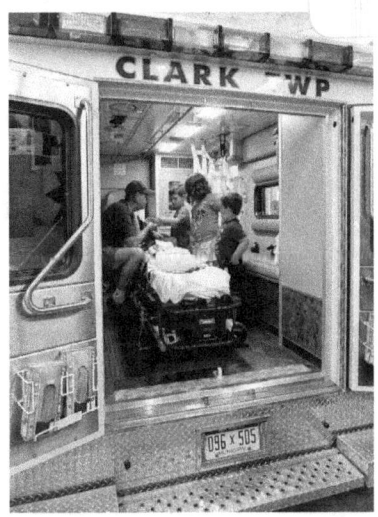

On Sept. 11, 2001, thousands of first responders
heroically rushed to the scene and saved
tens of thousands of lives.
More than 400 of those first responders
did not make it out alive.
In rushing into those burning buildings,
not one of them asked,
'What God do you pray to?'
What beliefs do you hold?'

Michael Bloomberg

Copyright 2018 by Dr. George Lindenfeld.
All rights reserved.

The right of Dr. George Lindenfeld to be identified as the author of this work is asserted by him in accordance with the Copyright, Designs and Patent's Act of 1988.

No part of this book may be reproduced in any form or by any electronic or mechanical means, including information storage and retrieval systems, except in the case of brief quotations embodied in critical articles or reviews, without permission in writing from the author in accordance with the Copyright, Designs and Patent's Act of 1988.

No portion of the material in this book is intended to offer personalized professional advice. This is not a self-help book. The information contained herein cannot replace or substitute for the service of a trained and licensed professional in the mental health field, including and limited to, licensed practitioners.

The author specifically disclaims any liability, loss or risk, personal or otherwise, that is incurred as a consequence, directly or indirectly, of the use and application of any of the content of this book.

Contents:

Contents............................5

Who Is This Book For?..................7

Foreword 11

Reflections 17

Acknowledgements 29

Introduction 31

Chapter 1   Whatever Doesn't Kill Us 35

Chapter 2   Policing 75

Chapter 3   Firefighting 117

Chapter 4   Emergency Medical Tech 155

Chapter 5   Emergency Nursing 183

Chapter 6   Emergency Physician 219

Chapter 7 Dispatcher/Telecommunicator . 251

Chapter 8 Correction Officer 283

Chapter 9 The Storm 349

Chapter 10 The Healing Sound 381

Epilogue 399

Who is this book for?

In my first book, *Ending the Nightmare of PTSD*, I chose to focus on our combat veterans and their significant others. I did this in order to instill a seed of hope where before, there has been prevailing despair. My intent was to inform our service men and women as well as their loved ones, that there now exists a rapid and noninvasive way to end the daily suffering incurred as a result of their combat related sacrifices. I chose to do this to replace the pervasive and erroneous belief that too many of our mental health professionals have about PTSD being a lifelong psychic injury that cannot be healed.

I perceive that first responders experience similar types of exposure to trauma that tend to have a cumulative effect over the course of a career. However, within the varied occupations that constitute this group, there are no rotations home related to their service. Nor are there national statistics acquired to determine their mental health status over the course of their employment.

Much like their comparative military cohorts, their exposure to traumatic situations comes home with them negatively. This tends to alter the quality of life of those who are close to them as well. Many opt out of their chosen professions due to burnout or as others call it, 'compassion fatigue'. Call it what you will, when it is trauma induced, I call it Post-Traumatic Stress (PTS).

My perspective is that human beings have not yet adapted to a level necessary for them to sustain the pressures and stresses of modern life. Rather, when we human-kind experience trauma, our minds are programmed at a genetic level to go into a defensive, protective mode to ensure our survival.

The relatively recent understanding of this self-protective cortical mechanism permits us to turn the growth switch back on later by resetting the altered and frozen neuronal circuitry. I have found that the switch can be reset even after a 50-year period, such as emotional trauma sustained initially in the Vietnam war era. My plan with this book is to address different first responder professions that are frequently exposed to PTS. I didn't plan on it at the time but, my ninth chapter describes first responders at their best when dealing with an oncoming natural disaster.

Within my research efforts related to combat veterans, I was stunned by the concurrence and elevated percentages of sleep disorders, nightmares and emergence of intimacy issues in those with chronic PTSD. Amazingly, this was the case even in those Veterans who were alleged to have 'successfully' completed treatment for trauma-related issues. How can we be so blind?

I've come to the conclusion that unless sleep disorder and nightmares as well as other comorbid issues are fully eliminated through the specified 'gold standard' or experimental treatment, the PTSD neuronal network remains activated, even if this is at a subconscious level.

Sustaining the mental wellness of our first-responders is critical in meeting our community's long-term needs. Unfortunately, the prevalent notion is that once traumatized, burnt out or afflicted with compassion fatigue through cumulative traumatic incidents, the damage is irreversible.

My research and therapeutic intervention with combat veterans suggests that this is absolute nonsense. We can reset our valued personnel to full functioning rapidly and through non-invasive means. This can be accomplished without chemicals or lengthy psychotherapy. This book has been written for the explicit purpose of bringing this knowledge into full and complete awareness. Furthermore, the data provided within each chapter clarifies the terrible toll that cumulative exposure to trauma has on the emotional and physical wellbeing of those who are there to protect us.

Foreword

Post-traumatic stress disorder (PTSD) is a terrible affliction that affects fire fighters and paramedics at double the rate of the general population, and is an ever-growing problem in all ranks of the fire service – one in five fire fighters/paramedics will suffer from PTSD in the course of their career, and those with PTSD are six times more likely to commit suicide.

While it's always existed, PTSD is just beginning to become more widely recognized as a major issue in the fire service. In fact, the hidden struggle with PTSD is one of the biggest threats to the health and security of our fire fighters.

Often, the stigma associated with asking for help prevents many in the fire service from admitting something is wrong. Even though trauma is a daily occurrence for fire fighters – most can recall with ease at least three horrific or tragic calls – they keep their behavioral health issues inside, worrying it will hurt their pride or reputation. But if left untreated, it only gets worse, destroying lives, families and careers.

So, we can no longer overlook or ignore behavioral health issues as "part of the job." Whether it's the unrelenting grip of PTSD, a life devastated by alcohol and drugs or the finality of suicide, we are losing too many of our own.

We have an obligation to make sure we provide every path possible to help these men and women recover from post-traumatic stress and the damage it can do to their lives and families. And every fire department has a role to play – from increasing awareness from day one at recruit school on behavioral health issues and offering coping and prevention strategies, to building peer support teams and providing continued education for fire fighters and fire chiefs.

While quality behavioral healthcare is available in many communities, it's not always effective for helping fire fighters and paramedics. We know from our members that even those who are courageous enough to ask for help aren't receiving treatment from mental health professionals who understand the unique culture and experiences of the fire service.

That's why it's important for fire fighters and the behavioral health community to work together in a systematic approach to not only fight stigma, but develop alternatives to the traditional behavioral health services and interventions available.

One such pioneer leading the fight to develop quality and culturally competent treatment for our fire fighters is Dr. George Lindenfeld, noted psychologist and accomplished author. In his fifth work, **First Responders: Compassion Fatigue, Burnout, & PTSD**, Dr. Lindenfeld dives deeply into the unique experiences of PTSD among the brave men and women who put their lives on the line every day to serve our communities.

Building on his expertise in treating active military and veteran populations who suffer from PTSD, Dr. Lindenfeld has developed a promising new intervention that uses sensory activation to reconsolidate traumatic memories without relying on the traditional talk therapy interventions that in some cases have been ineffective or even a deterrent for those seeking help.

I am grateful for Dr. Lindenfeld's contribution to bring the critical issues of PTSD in the fire service to the forefront of our national and international awareness. We have an uphill battle to climb in addressing this crisis among our ranks, but when we work together to challenge versus accept what is, we are one step closer.

Sincerely,

Harold A. Schaitberger
General President
International Association of Firefighters

Harold Schaitberger, General President of the International Association of Fire Fighters, began his career as a professional fire fighter in Fairfax County, Virginia. He quickly rose to the rank of lieutenant, organized and served as president of his local and the Virginia Professional Fire Fighters – all before he had seven years on the job.

Before becoming General President, he headed the IAFF's political and legislative operation for nearly 25 years.

During his tenure as General President, he has demonstrated an unbending commitment to ensure the health, safety and security of IAFF members and their families. Under his leadership, he has ensured that the IAFF is at the forefront in addressing health issues in the fire service, including cancer and behavioral health, devoting resources to preventing and treating cancer – which is scientifically proven to occur in fire fighters at higher rates than the general population – as well as push for presumptive protections. And, the IAFF is leading efforts to help members struggling with post-traumatic stress and other behavioral health issues, including opening the IAFF Center of Excellence for Behavioral Health Treatment and Recovery, specifically for fire fighters.

The International Association of Fire Fighters is the driving force behind nearly every advance in the fire and emergency services in the 21st century. With headquarters in Washington, DC, and Ottawa, Ontario, the IAFF represents more than 310,000 full-time professional fire fighters and paramedics in more than 3,200 affiliates in the United States and Canada.

Reflections:

Reading Dr. Lindenfeld's chapter on emergency medicine, I am reminded of the exhilaration I felt sitting in the back of the flying squad ambulance, sirens wailing as we rushed to deal with a woman having a post-partum hemorrhage. And then, there was my terror confronting a desperately sick child in the emergency room. In both these scenarios, as a junior intern, I felt very inadequately trained to deal with the task at hand but this was not atypical for its time – the late 1960's. Emergency medicine is a specialty field now and yet, despite all the advances, the corporatization of medicine presents a huge threat to quality of care and to the well-being of those tasked with providing this essential service.

Lindenfeld vividly describes the stress and trauma and burnout of the typical emergency room physician. He does not exaggerate – surveys have shown that a high percentage of medical students suffer burnout and suicidal ideation; this even before graduation. Unhealthy patterns of lifestyle are set up and continue throughout the career. He rightfully points out the tragedy of burnout, drug addiction and suicide – all well-recognized occupational hazards, known about for many years.

I find the chapter on the emergency physician to be a well-researched and a well-written treatise having application not only in the ER setting but to the medical profession in general. It is my hope that it will serve as a wake-up call to the unrelenting drama, daily stress and poor nourishment for the spirit that accompanies the physician's challenge to do no harm to those who seek his/her expertise.

It is my perspective that the creation of a healthcare system that fosters and supports the enlightened physician would require radical institutional change from medical school training to retirement; tough to imagine in this era of corporatization of medicine. Until this is undertaken, what are we to do with the walking wounded – the professionals who have been traumatized - even to the extent of some suffering from PTSD? In my role of physician mentor, I have assisted a number of these physicians while their cries for help have been dismissed or gone unheard.

George Lindenfeld has heard their cries and responded with his RESET program - one of a number of emerging alternative medicine interventions. Perhaps interventions of this type may assist these impaired professionals to enhance rather than suppress their own sense of inner awareness. While the problems facing the medical community remain multifactorial, **any** action step that has the potential to facilitate a more balanced life for those interested in the occupation of medicine, is to be welcomed and fully endorsed.

Barry Bub, MD
Author Communication Skills that Heal,
A Practical Approach to a New Professionalism
in Medicine (Radcliffe 2006)

"There are many days after I leave work, that I come home and ask my husband, 'Why do I continue to do this?' Running throughout the emergency room, mindlessly completing tasks that the doctors ordered, taking patients to the restroom and putting them on the bedpan, getting them a certain requested snack, giving the drug seeking patient the longed for IV opioid they've requested. I frequently joke about an R.N. being a 'refreshment and narcotic' nurse, because sometimes that's what it feels like.

"I can't agree more with the term, 'I love emergency nursing, but I hate people.' It is hard to work in such a high-demand environment and not become biased towards the general population. I was triaging patients in our fast track just the other day when I called up this gentleman, assumingly for 'foot pain.' I said, 'sir what brings you into the emergency department today?' He says, 'I'm on blood thinners and a bunch of otha' heart meds.' I responded, 'OK sir, but what brings you in TODAY' He repeats his medications to me. Becoming frustrated at this point, I said 'Sir, I don't care about your medications right now, I am trying to figure out why you came to the emergency room today.' He then proceeded to call me rude and told me to read his chart. Growing more agitated, and knowing his main complaint was foot pain due to the intake process we have at our hospital, I put in his note, 'Pt. to the ED with c/o Foot pain. Pt. told me to read his chart, and that he is on a blood thinner. Pt. not answering any other questions at this time.' Shortly after another patient came up to me as I was with another patient, demanding stronger pain medicine as the ones they gave her, 'weren't doing shit.' I eagerly charted in her chart with her statement in exact quotes, just because. As these episodes kept happening in the fast track this particular day, it was an, 'I truly hate people day.'

"Growing up in a medical family, I wanted to be a nurse for as long as I remember. My mom always told me how great a career it was. After getting into it, I have come to the realization that it is truly a thankless job. We work long 12+ hour shifts with most days escaping for five minutes to run to the cafeteria for some food. All too often we are inhaling our sandwich at the desk, and looking up to see a family member, requesting that their loved one be placed on a bedpan.

Unfortunately, the medical field has turned into a business. With Medicare payments now depending on HCAHPS (Hospital Consumer Assessment of Healthcare Providers and Systems) scores to determine the amount of paying their hospital, our hospital is trained on providing 'patient care with a smile.' It is crazy to believe that those who sit in offices all day care more about patient satisfaction rather than nurse burn out and nurse dissatisfaction.

"Specifically, at my hospital, our management is very supportive and backs the staff 150% with unruly patients. However, one can only assume it is not like that everywhere. Getting into nursing itself, I thought it would be rainbows and butterflies like in the movies. You would treat patients medically and do what is necessary for their healing. Now it has turned into worrying about how they score you on a survey afterwards. The nursing shortage in 2018 does not make nursing easier. As you wish 100% of your staff were hardworking team players, they never are.

Some days I feel like I am running around with a bunch of sick patients, while looking over at my coworker texting. It is nice when you come into work with your favorite staff members and can breathe a sigh of relief and think no matter how hard the day may be, your staff rocks.

ER nursing is a whole new beast. One of the HCAHPS survey questions is 'how your pain is controlled.' A lot of the time, pain is acute sending a majority of the patients into the ER looking for pain relief. This specific issue automatically triggers an ER nurse's brain to think, 'drug seeker.' Although we try not to make these assumptions and change our plan of care, as soon as we even think about the patient being a drug seeker, our behavior changes. We visit the patient less often, we medicate as little as we can, and we are inclined to write that patient off. This is because we become numb to pain seeking individuals. As frequent as it is, you do the least amount for those people that may need it the most.

"As flu season is upon us, with low staffing and high census, I find myself running around with no lunch breaks and having to deal with a truly sick population. The burn out discussed in the book chapter is real, very real. My days off from work are usually spent at home and some days have to force myself to get out of bed. My feet ache, my back hurts. I do what I do because I love it. I love the adrenaline rush I get when we get in a trauma, or a code, or an unruly drunk or high patient that has to be restrained by four cops. There is never a day I don't go home absolutely exhausted both mentally and physically, but I can't imagine working anywhere else."

Alexandra Whitaker
Emergency Room R.N.

When I first entered the NYC Police Department, I was told that if I wanted to make it to retirement, I should avoid the three B's – bribes; booze and broads. I pretty much followed that advice and indeed, it really worked out that way. Twelve years into my career, I was assigned to a special unit called Special Operations Division (SOD). The mission of this unit was to be able to respond to varied circumstances including terrorist attacks. I was trained in heavy weapon use as well as cross trained as an EMT to be able to assist in those circumstances where immediate medical assistance was necessary.

Experience has taught me that the worse a precinct is, the more bonded one becomes to ones' comrades because you need to back each other up. Also, I've noticed that the firemen in such a precinct are also much closer. For the most part, I have found that officers that were developing emotional difficulties weren't very forthcoming. You really don't want to hear that your partner is in a weakened state and can't back you up.

I remember a particular situation where my partner and I were chasing a perp and he collapsed and I thought he was taking a heart attack. I took him to the ER and the doc there brought him a paper bag and told him to breathe into it, because he had been hyperventilating. Things like that were embarrasssing so we dealt with it by not talking about it.

With the code, anyone who makes a little noise is going to get attention. You don't want attention! They have a big book called the Rules & Procedures and they'll find something in there to quiet the noise. The basic message is that you come to work, do your job, and keep your mouth shut. It's the camaraderie that you want to maintain.

With administration, I didn't like giving out tickets so they reassigned me to a precinct that required me to pay a toll every time I came to work and went home. There didn't seem to be too much empathy forthcoming at that level to those of us who served on the line.

I served in an area referred to as an A-House, which is one of the worst crime areas in the city. Of course, in those kind of circumstances, we tended to deal with people in different ways. In my district, we had one square mile with three hundred police officers assigned. Even in that context, we had about one hundred homicides a year.

During my service, I almost lost my own life on three occasions. I vividly recall one in which we were ordered to the scene of a murder and while attending to the body in front of a tenement, someone on the roof dropped a huge sewer cover that nearly hit me. Looking up with my weapon drawn, all I could see were numerous people looking out of their windows. That one really shook me up! Stuff like that is a little scary. I buried these thoughts a long time ago but candidly, as I bring them up again, the emotional part of it is still there.

With police suicide, in my time, officers didn't discuss their emotional matters and were more inclined to keep it in, suppress it. I recall one officer who had plenty of money, everything seemed fine, and one day, just before his retirement, he blew his brains out. They said he was suffering from depression but he never showed it or talked about it. On the other side of the coin, over the years, I saved at least seven or so people's lives in different settings. Being a police officer means that you are never truly off duty. I continue to feel that way today even though I've been retired for years.

Ole Olsen
New York City Police Officer - retired

Following my read of the firefighters' chapter, I realize that I still miss the adrenaline rush related to my 25 years of service. It all began after my assignment to Engine 58 in Harlem, NYC on fifth Avenue around 115th St. We were like number three in the city in runs and number one in structural, occupied work. Later, I was assigned to Rockaway to a company called Ladder 521. Over time, I worked in every borough except Staten Island.

Early on, I was told that there were collapses but that tenement buildings didn't do that. We were stretching up the interior staircase of a tenement and it felt like the whole building rocked and rolled. Thank God we had the radios on because I said to be careful - the whole back of the building collapsed while we were in it.

I recall one time being the second unit to a fire, and later, we walked into the actual fire room. There on the floor was a little skeleton of a little infant. That was pretty shocking! It was a hard one to put out of my head.

Regarding drinking, early when I went in, there was a great deal of it but my understanding is that later, it wasn't tolerated and people were released from service if it continued. A couple of guys I knew had heart attacks but I'm not sure if that was due to congenital factors or to the job. I don't think my body really got used to shift work even though what

I was at it for 25 years. I really think in retrospect that it's a young man's job!

I went to visit my daughter in Washington, DC two years after I retired and I didn't know that there was a fire house across the street from her. In the middle of the night, the fire station doors opened and an air horn started going off and I jumped out of bed and started immediately putting my clothes on. It was like Pavlov's response! Like it was still in my muscle memory. Guess that my training and experiences will never leave me.

After retirement, we always had reunions and stuff giving the guys the opportunity to come back and talk with each other about what bothered us. We did little talking outside of that circle sparing our families from what we had to deal with often on a daily basis. It was years after my retirement that I found out that my career really upset my daughter. I remember her telling me, when she was a child, that she didn't like me going off to work. She was afraid that I wouldn't come back. As far as the marriage, I'm sure it affected it but I really liked my job and it was a steady paycheck although my wife thought I was kind of crazy to continue doing it. We really never talked much about it. If I was younger, I would still want to do it. I miss the rush, camaraderie, all of it!

Anomymous
New York City Fireman - retired

Acknowledgements:

There have been so many who have contributed to this book either directly or indirectly. Those who have shared their personal stories and experiences through varied venues, deserve to be acknowledged. By discussing their own personal tragedies, they have become heroes in their own right. They have done so in order to forewarn others regarding the perils of cumulative stress.

I will begin with my heartfelt appreciation to Harold A. Schaitberger, General President of the International Association of Firefighters. His recognition of the critical issues of PTSD within the fire service is certainly to be considered a formal recognition of the ongoing challenges these public servants face. By breaking down the walls that block firefighters from access to newly available remediative interventions, he takes a leap into the future wherein restorative possibilities replace the cumulative and far too often deadly effects of stress.

An honorable mention is provided to Brigadier General James Hesson, who steadfastly supported and mentored me in my efforts to gain community and national support for our much-needed exploration of remediative interventions.

I extend my appreciation to Dr. Frank Lawlis for his creation of the BAUD as well as the basic protocols leading to the emerging development of RESET Therapy.

My appreciation continues for my colleague, Dr. George Rozelle, for providing his 'Brian Mapping' expertise within the context of our research efforts. This extends further to other enduring members of our team including: Dr. James Miller and Dr. Michael Sutherland. I also express my appreciation to Donna Iraneta for proofing the entirety of this book. I have come to call Donna the comma queen as clearly, I didn't learn this skill properly within my early education.

To those who contributed to my 'Reflections Section' including: Anonymous - New York City Fireman - retired; Dr. Barry Bub, Family Physician – retired; Ole Olsen, New York City Policeman – Retired; Alexandra Whitaker - Emergency Room R.N., I thank you so much for taking the time to reflect on how your selective chapter resonated with your own professional experience.

Finally, I extend my thanks to those first responders who have chosen a career of committed service to our communities and to our nation. This book is dedicated to those who provide such service in order to keep us well and safe from harm. They in turn, deserve the best from us to protect them from the traumas they face too often.

Introduction:

The term **first responder** refers to those who have been trained to assist within the context of an emergency, whether it be due to natural causes, accidents or terrorist inspired events. Certified first responders have received specialized training and passed a competency exam qualifying them to provide pre-hospital care for medical emergencies.

Within the context of emergency situations, licensed personnel such as emergency room nurses and physicians have received extensive training prior to their service. These specialists may have first contact with those who are injured or, they may receive those who are injured transported to them by firefighters, police officers, paramedics or others, such as family members.

Typically, those who make a choice to become first responders are emotionally stable individuals. However, over the course of their service and consequent exposure to ongoing stress and episodic trauma, a shift may occur altering the individual in a negative manner.

Within the military, the term **'suck it up and truck on'** implies that one's own needs are secondary to the purpose and mission of the unit. There is no equivalent statement among the diverse group composing first responders that I know of, particularly with some aspects of these collective service providers being primarily male (firefighters) while others (nurses) are primarily female.

Within each specialty, I'm sure that there exists expectation of behavior equivalent to **'man up'** that implies disdain for the evidencing of signs of weakness in regard to one's mental status. Indeed, if one were to risk sharing information of this type with a colleague, this may result in scorn and disparagement. Thus, the cumulative effects of stress, including exposure to traumatic events, are inclined to be kept internal and compartmentalized.

The unspoken code requires the individual to suppress inner discomfort, for to evidence it is seen by others as a sign of weakness and probable character defect. The customary means of coping with these matters are certainly available, such as using alcohol to neutralize the accumulating effects of stress. In fact, this is best done among others in the group in order to sustain the camaraderie that is necessary for unit cohesion.

This mix of acceptable and unacceptable behaviors directs the individual along a path leading to conflicted functioning, often reducing the effectiveness and efficiency of the afflicted individual. Ultimately, the acquired means of coping begins to fail.

Human nature as it is, suggests that when something isn't working any longer, do what worked previously even harder. Thus, if alcohol was the solution, do this even more. Ultimately, the body becomes unable to sustain the effects of 'burning the candle at both ends.' It is at this point where symptoms become evident because they can no longer be suppressed.

Overcoming the 'code,' indeed is a challenging task. And yet, to maintain the effectiveness of the unit as a whole, it is necessary to take a 'top down' look at the system that is currently in place. With 'sanction' for alternative solutions to address the cumulative effects of stress and trauma, it is my hope that gradually the system will change.

My purpose in writing this book is to apply what I have learned from our combat veterans with PTSD to those first responders who have experienced a parallel effect referred to as compassion fatigue.

Based on new neuroscientific advances, we now know with certainty that it is possible to return the afflicted individual to a state of enhanced functioning, both physically, mentally and spiritually. The restoration of hope for this potential is my primary objective in writing this book.

I truly believe that the 'code' can be adapted to better meet the needs of the unit as well as the unique individual needs of each of its members. Furthermore, by re-stabilizing the individual, other family members of the first responder may also be provided with the opportunity to recover from the 'secondary effects' of their exposure to 'compassion fatigue.'

Chapter One

"Whatever doesn't kill us makes us stronger"

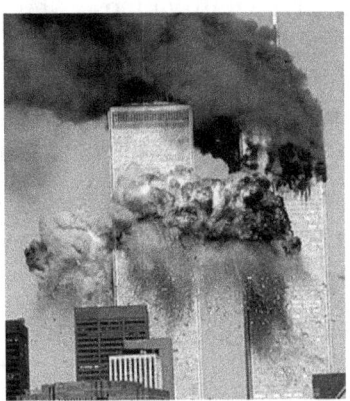

Remember the hours after September 11th when we came together as one to answer the attack against our homeland. We drew strength when our firefighters ran upstairs and risked their lives so that others might live; when rescuers rushed into smoke and fire at the Pentagon; when the men and women of Flight 93 sacrificed themselves to save our Nation's Capital; when flags were hanging from front porches all across America, and strangers became friends. It was the worst day we have ever seen, but it brought out the best in all of us.

Senator John Kerry

"9/11/2001 was a day in which innocence was lost to the American public. The reality of trauma and its aftermath in the form of Post-Traumatic Stress Disorder, as well as numerous medical complications due to environmental factors, came rushing head-on to confront those who were directly involved in it.

"In the aftermath of the 9/11 attack, 2,996 persons were killed and 6,000 plus persons were wounded. Specifically, 2,606 perished at the World Trade Center (WTC) and surrounding area. 265 died on the four planes and 125 died at the Pentagon.

"343 Firefighters and 71 Law Enforcement personnel perished at the WTC. At the Pentagon, 55 military personnel lost their lives. 2,135 U.S. civilians died in the attacks while 372 non-U.S. individuals representing more than 90 countries perished as well.

". . . It has been reported that over 1,400, 9/11 rescue workers who responded to the scene in the days and months after the attacks have since died. At least ten unborn babies also died on 9/11." ("Lower Manhattan," 2016)

On this day, our trust and sense of safety was seriously weakened. A shock wave of fear rippled across the nation. We were at war, but with whom? The aftereffects of 9/11 continue into the present.

Please note that varied investigators are referring to the aftereffects from this cataclysmic experience as PTSD. Researchers have investigated nearly one-fifth of WTC responders, half of whom still have active PTSD disorder 11–13 years later.

They noted that: "The most frequent symptoms in the active PTSD group were avoidance and hyperarousal symptoms, while intrusive recollection symptoms were less commonly endorsed. . . More than a decade after 9/11, WTC exposures remained strongly predictive of both active and remitted PTSD, especially among police responders.

". . . The percentage with post-9/11 PTSD in our sample (17.7%) and the weighted percentage for the entire WTCHP (18.2%) are consistent with the lifetime rate of 18.7% in the National Vietnam Veterans Readjustment Study (NVVRS) theater cohort assessed with the SCID 20–25 years later." (Dohrenwend, Turner, Turse, Lewis-Fernandez, & Yager, 2008)

The findings from the above study are profound, suggesting that combat veterans with PTSD and 9/11 exposed individuals experience close to the same rate of PTSD symptomology. Yet another study reported that: ". . . although the diagnosis of PTSD connotes 'flashbacks' and 'nightmares' in popular culture, these symptoms were far less frequently reported than avoidance and hyperarousal symptoms. "Furthermore, the trajectory of PTSD symptoms among responders with active PTSD showed progressively increasing symptom severity, indicating both unmet need for treatment and potential under-treatment for those receiving mental health services.

"Although 'gold standard' treatments, such as cognitive–behavioral therapy and prolonged exposure therapy, were designed to address PTSD symptoms, a meta-analysis (Watts et al., 2013), showed that these treatments potentially benefit only one in two patients." (Huffman, Niazi, Rundell, Sharpe, & Katon, 2014)

A more recent (2016) article noted that: "The concurrent associations with poorer health and psychosocial well-being were striking, particularly for responders with active PTSD though the remitted group also had a 2-fold increased level of dissatisfaction with life and negative subjective health." (Bromet et al., 2016)

By remitted, I perceive that the authors are referring to the absence of active symptoms associated with the PTSD condition. Alternatively, 'dissatisfaction with life' and 'negative subjective health' clearly does not suggest that the afflicted individuals have returned to the life status that they had previously experienced. Indeed, many perceive that once an individual has experienced a major traumatic event such as 9/11, they will never be the same.

I'd like to offer an opinion on the topic of spontaneous long-term remission. As discussed in my 2016 book: *PTSD Comorbid Conditions Including: Addiction; Chronic Pain; Complex PTSD; Dementia; Depression; Sleep Disorder; Survivor's Guilt; Traumatic Brain Injury*, Delayed Onset Post-Traumatic Stress Disorder (DOPTSD) is emerging as an issue of concern among our aging veterans. The suggestion here is that the symptoms can become dormant over decades as opposed to being totally and completely extinguished.

To add further to this matter, a recent 2017 study explored the relationship between C-Reactive Protein (CRP) which is considered to be a marker of systemic inflammation, with scores for PTSD. The researchers found that: "In this large study of the relationship between CRP and posttraumatic stress pathology, we demonstrated an association between systemic inflammation and stress pathology (PTSD; trending with depression), which remained after adjusting for potentially confounding variables.

"These results contribute to research findings suggesting a salient relationship between inflammation and posttraumatic stress pathology." (Rosen et al., 2017)

Emerging data of this type is authenticating the perception that the symptoms of PTSD, and might I add compassion fatigue, go beyond psychological manifestations and rather, effect the mind, body and spirit as a whole.

Before we delve further into issues associated with being a first responder, I'd like to inform you of a tradition I've developed in my writing of prior books. From time to time within each chapter, I will insert personal anecdotes from first responders. I do this to bring to your awareness the plight of these at-risk personnel and indeed, this at-risk profession.

Because of the length of some of these testaments, I've condensed some material trying to keep in pertinent comments. Where there are grammatical errors, I've left them unchanged. Each anecdote will have a line of asterisks before and after and will be indented within this special space.

A number of the stories I've provided can be accessed through the Code Green Campaign that was founded in March of 2014 by a group of EMS professionals. This occurred after they became aware of the high rate of Post-Traumatic Stress Disorder and suicide among first responders.

As this is still a relatively young organization reaching out to a variety of first responders, the preponderance of their material is from the EMS community. I extrapolate this data to all first responders within the context of the stories provided. The Code Green was initially founded as a storytelling project and can be accessed at: http://codegreen-campaign.org/.

****

16.100: I am a 18 plus year EMT. I don't know if I have PTSD, i don't know how that mental pain is measured. I know I suffer from mental illness, some of it personal and some of it professional. I have thought of suicide, I have attempted suicide, and times I have wished I was brave enough to follow through or lucky enough to have completed it. I've seen councillors, I've seen psychologists, I've even spent a week in a mental institute.

. . . I've self medicated with alcohol and misused prescription medications. I've talked to family, I've talked to colleagues but mostly I've suffered alone. I am ashamed of my mental illness, I'm ashamed that I'm not a better EMT or human being. My self loathing knows no bounds. But I continue to come to work. I put on my poker face and hide what I truly think and feel. I don't even cry anymore.

. . . My councilor calls it "empathy burnout". I can tell she hesitates to tell me honestly I might never get that level of empathy back. I could quit. But then what? I've done this so long I don't know anything else. I don't have faith in myself to learn anything else. I'm too old to start over. I'm a failure but I've managed to fool everyone around me. They all say I'm a good EMT, I have high praise from my supervisor. No one knows I'm a fake.

Story written by an anonymous EMT 18 years in EMS.

****

A 2011 European Agency for Safety and Health at Work (EU-OSHA) article provided us with a comprehensive view of what is occurring worldwide as a consequence of natural and manmade disasters that include the following scenarios: "everyday emergencies (road accidents, crime scenes, gas explosions, fires); natural disasters (floods, storms, fires, earthquakes, volcanic eruptions); industrial accidents (involving hazardous materials, such as in the nuclear and mining sectors); transport accidents (major car crashes, plane crashes, rail accidents); terrorist and criminal attacks (bomb attacks, gas attacks, shootings); massive public events (negative events during concerts, sport events, demonstrations)."

The authors further noted that: "In the last 25 years, the psychological trauma suffered by emergency and rescue workers has gained the attention of scientists. Although studies show that the majority of rescue workers may experience stress that does not necessarily lead to diagnosable mental disorders, a variety of symptoms such as strong emotional reactions (shock, anger, guilt, helplessness), cognitive reactions (disorientation, lack of concentration), physical reactions (tension, fatigue, pain, racing heartbeat) and social effects (isolation from family and friends) may for some time after an incident have a negative impact on workers' wellbeing.

"More serious problems such as acute stress disorder, depression, anxiety, and post-traumatic stress disorders have also been diagnosed. A Swedish study indicates a prevalence of between

3% and 25% of PTSD among rescue workers there." ("!2013-3rded-advocacyhandbook-interactive. pdf," 2013)

****

I've been struggling to convince the man I love (30+ years as a Police Officer) to seek help for his PTSD; however, it has been to no avail. He's exhibiting many of the symptoms mentioned here. I just don't know what to say or do to convince/persuade him to seek professional help. My heart breaks to see him suffer and know that he is self medicating with alcohol. The murders, fatal car accidents, suicides, domestic violence and most recently, one of the first responders to his dear friend/retired police officer's suicide is consuming him.

Story written by an anonymous first responder's spouse.

****

I find the use of the term 'Remitted PTSD,' as discussed earlier, to be quite interesting. Looking into this further, I accessed Google Search and came up with four hits including the following information: "Post-traumatic stress disorder has also been found to be associated with a reduced capacity for reward processing. Male Vietnam veterans with PTSD reported lower reward expectancies and lower satisfaction with received reward compared to male Vietnam veterans without PTSD when performing a wheel of fortune-type gambling task." (Hopper et al., 2008).

Using the same task, Elman et al. noted that: ". . . These blunted responses to rewards have been related to the symptoms of 'emotional numbing' observed in PTSD that include diminished interest in significant activities, feelings of detachment from others, and restricted range of affect." (Elman et al., 2005), American Psychiatric Association, (Association, 2013)

So, what are we to make of this new term called Remitted PTSD? Does it mean that even in the absence of glaring PTSD symptomology, the best mental health professionals can do is to offer a life blunted from the world of emotions? Is it our goal to produce results that induce: "emotional numbing observed in PTSD that include diminished interest in significant activities, feelings of detachment from others, and restricted range of affect?" (Elman et al. 2005).

To this last question, I must respond with, "Hell no!" We can and will do better. We have the means to return the afflicted individual to pre-trauma levels. Yes, it needs to be evaluated and validated and is still considered to be experimental in nature. But, how can we settle for less? Those who have served, whether at home or abroad deserve, "the full Monty" (everything which is necessary, appropriate or possible; 'the works').

Next, I'd like to respond to the implications of the Rosen et. al., study. Systemic inflammation takes us beyond the realm of psychological symptoms. Inflammation is a self-protective, immune system reaction aimed at initiating the healing process by removing damaged cells, irritants, or pathogens. The speculation here is that damage occurs at both a cortical and physical level.

Consequently, the structure of this book is framed around the objective of fully and totally reversing PTSD/Compassion Fatigue symptomology stuck in the neuronal network of the brain and body. I will elucidate this intention in each chapter, building upon material I've provided in my earlier manuscripts. My plan for this introductory chapter is to refer to first responders as a unitary group. In later chapters, I will differentiate the varied specialties with their particular vulnerabilities and exposures to stress and environmental influences.

****

"16.102: As I sit here drinking my 6th scotch after many beers all I can think about is your son. . . I have nightmares about you begging me to save him. I want you to know there was absolutely. Nothing I could do. . . I sit here, depress with my last bit of strength. I absolutely hate my job and everything I do. I hate that I can't sleep. I hate that i could t help you in your time of need. I want to to k ow that your screams, your begging, your pleading, will forever replay in my mind. . . Please forgive me.

"Please understand there was nothing I could do. Please understand the reason I drink. Please understand my heartache. . . I absolutely hate my life, my career, my life choices. . . Please understand I will never forgive myself or the circumstances.

"Please know you and your son will always be with me. Please understand that I will never be the same, just like you. . . If it was up to me your baby boy would still be alive. Please know that while I continue tomorrow drink myself into this hole that you will forever be in my mind. Please know I'm truly sorry."

*Story written by an
anonymous first responder.*

****

I'll begin by describing the first responder's overall exposure to the: impact of ongoing stress; vulnerability to trauma; environmental hazards. I'll also discuss the presence of PTSD in this collective group as well as 'burnout' tendencies.

The authors of the following article compared first responders to military personnel advising us that: "First responders and military personnel face occupational exposures that have been associated with altered immune and inflammatory activity. In turn, these physiological responses are linked to altered moods and feelings of well-being which may provide priming conditions that compromise individual resilience and increase the risk of PTSD and depression when subsequently exposed to acute traumatic events.

"These exposures include heat, smoke, and sleep restriction, and physical injury often alongside heavy physical exertion. Provided the stimulus is sufficient, these exposures have been linked to inflammatory activity and modification of the hypothalamic–pituitary axis (HPA), offering a mechanism for the high rates of PTSD and depressive disorders in these occupations." (Walker, McKune, Ferguson, Pyne, & Rattray, 2016)

I'm unsure if the authors of the preceding article are suggesting that environmental exposure is the precursor to a weakened immune system which then renders the individual susceptible to the onset of PTSD. I do agree that both trauma and environmental exposure may lead to 'inflammatory activity.'

However, I also perceive that PTSD can 'ignite' systemically through an onslaught of traumatic exposure alone. Returning now to matters related to first responders, let's discuss how this profession is described in an informative recruitment article that follows: "First responders, officially called emergency medical responders as of January 1, 2012, (according to the National Registry of Emergency Medical Technicians), are the people who first arrive to help you after you've dialed 911 for emergency assistance.

"Once they are on the scene, first responders assess the situation, request additional help when necessary and provide basic first aid, which could include such duties as controlling hemorrhage, bandaging wounds, providing cardiopulmonary resuscitation (CPR), assisting in childbirth and taking care of general medical issues and emergencies.

"The first responder's goal is to provide basic, lifesaving interventions while waiting for additional emergency response assistance to arrive. In addition to providing medical care, first responders also work to stabilize the incident scene, protect property and, in cases of criminal activity, preserve evidence. The term 'first responder' refers to a level of emergency response training. People holding this title include firefighters, police officers, search and rescue professionals, emergency medical service workers and hazardous materials personnel, to name a few."
("Becoming a First responder: Job Description & Salary Info," 2017)

****

"16.98: Tonight is another sleepless night. I've tried all the old tricks. Took an Ambien and then a few hours later a Xanax, and yet I'm still wide awake. Feeling lonely, sad, and unimportant. Sometimes those emotions just show up, no prompts, no real drama and just slide to the front and I can't shake them. . .

"I do what I'm suppose to. I see the shrink. I answer his questions the way I'm suppose. I take my antidepressant religiously. I tell him I'm not suicidal but sometimes late at night I contemplate how much easier it would be to give up and give in to the utter despair.

"It never ends. It never goes away. You will yourself to fight. You lie to yourself and say it will get better. And maybe it will. . . for awhile. But then it's back. And everything hurts. And you just want it to end."

*anonymous flight paramedic
12 years in EMS.*

****

There is much research pertaining to personality variables that may help to insulate one from the effects of trauma. An example of such research is found in a 2000 article by Regher, et al., entitled: Individual Predictors of Traumatic Reactions in Firefighters. The authors refer to a trend for: ". . . theorists and researchers in the area of trauma (who) are pointing to the importance of individual differences in resilience and vulnerability as key determinants of the intensity and duration of trauma-related symptoms." (Regehr, Hill, & Glancy, 2000)

In my opinion, the exploration of personality aspects and how they may or may not influence the expression of PTSD symptomology begs the question. The underlying premise of this type of inquiry presupposes that ultimately, we will be able to develop a screening test to identify individuals who are more resilient to the cumulative effects of trauma.

In my mind, we are all potentially vulnerable when exposed to random or ongoing trauma simply because we are human beings whatever the personality type. I further believe that there is little question that ultimately, repeated exposure to trauma takes its destructive toll. Thus, at this point, I will express my own bias about risk and trauma as elucidated in my book entitled: *The Treatment of PTSD Comorbid Conditions Including: Addiction; Chronic Pain; Complex PTSD; Dementia; Depression; Sleep Disorder; Survivor's Guilt, Traumatic Brain Injury.*

In referring to the Regehr, et al., text that discussed the trait of resilience, I referenced the emergence of Delayed Onset Post-Traumatic Stress Disorder. This has been found to occur among our aging veteran population as noted in the first chapter in my PTSD Comorbid Conditions book. I also postulated that unless primary signs of the ongoing presence of

PTSD are fully eliminated, such as insomnia and nightmares, the trauma altered brain network remains intact.

This trauma altered circuit doesn't depend upon 'will of character' or for that matter, other personality variables. It is rather, a systemic reaction to a triggering event or series of events that alters overall functioning of the afflicted individual to some degree or other.

Whether it is expressed immediately or bubbles in the slow cooker located in the emotional center of the brain, it has the potential to negatively impact those who experience it. It is my position that the network must be reset to pre-trauma levels to restore normative growth and functioning.

****

"Facebook Post: PTSD for Firefighters is real. If your love one is experiencing signs get them help quickly. 27 years of deaths and babies dying in your hands is a memory that you will never get rid off. It haunted me daily until now. My love to my crews. Be safe , take care. I love you all.

"INDIAN RIVER COUNTY — Firefighters and paramedics are mourning the death of a man who worked alongside them for nearly three decades.

"Indian River County Sheriff deputies went to a wooded area off State Road 60 west of Interstate 95 about 10:30 p.m. Saturday following a 911 call from Indian River County Fire Rescue Battalion Chief David Dangerfield, Sheriff's spokesman Lt. Eric Flowers said.

"Dangerfield had driven his pickup to mile marker 13 about midway between I-95 and Yeehaw Junction, Flowers said. Dangerfield told dispatchers where he could be found, Flowers said. Deputies located the pickup and found Dangerfield a short distance away in the woods, dead from a self-inflicted gunshot wound, the Sheriff's Office said.

"Emergency Services Director John King sent an email late Saturday night to Dangerfield's co-workers about his death, Assistant Chief Brian Burkeen said.

"'It is with great sadness I share with you the passing of Battalion Chief David Dangerfield this evening,'

King wrote in the email to his firefighters and paramedics. "Please keep Dave's immediate and extended family in your thoughts and prayers ("Veteran IRC firefighter commits suicide shortly after PTSD post on Facebook |Photos, 2016")."

****

The topic of suicide among our first responders is difficult to ascertain. In comparison to the way that the CDC maintains its records, some of our states preserve data that is illuminating in regard to first responder deaths.

The following study investigated this occurrence from the periods of 2004 to 2011 with the following results forthcoming: ". . . due to the nature of their occupation, first responders are exposed to a number of violent situations and traumatic or stressful events that may increase their risk for violent death. The purpose of this study was to examine violent deaths among first responders using data collected by the North Carolina Violent Death Reporting System.

". . . In North Carolina between 2004 and 2011, 75 law enforcement officers, 23 firefighters, and 19

EMS personnel died as a result of violence. Of these deaths, 74% were suicides and 22% were homicides. . . All of the violent deaths among EMS personnel were the result of suicide, and the majority of homicide deaths were among law enforcement officers with 52% occurring while the officer was on duty." ("0017 Violent deaths among first responders: using north carolina violent death reporting system data to inform injury programs -- Austin et al. 21 (Suppl 1): A6 -- Injury Prevention," 2015)

As a next step in my exploration of suicidal ideation and enactment among our first responders, I looked into the review of literature pertaining to this topic. A 2016 examination investigated a number of studies on this topic. The authors found that: ". . . In this systematic review, we present 63 quantitative studies examining suicidal thoughts, behaviors, and/or fatalities among first responders; . . . Findings reveal elevated risk for suicide among first responders." (Stanley, Hom, & Joiner, 2016)

I acknowledge that the topic of suicide among our first responders, to state it politely, has been poorly investigated. Why can't bureaucracy, such as the CDC, target and tag occupations that are presently listed in varied categories so that we can obtain credible national data about the extent of death through suicide among our first responders?

I find it necessary to comment on why this focus on suicide is so critical in motivating the 'powers that be' to implement real solutions rather than perpetuating interventions that have been shown to be relatively ineffective. Our national focus on 20 veteran deaths per day due to suicide is the reason. When we have a hard number that our communities can rally around, real change can begin.

Furthermore, my intent in discussing this topic is to: lay a foundation of hope among our dispirited first responders rather than one of ongoing despair; of a life with meaning rather than a longing for death; of a future of public service by skilled and committed personnel rather than an isolative existence leading to despair, with thoughts and acts of self-destruction.

****

"14.20: Message: ****In Loving Memory of Carlos Lopez**** I went to Paramedic school with Carlos over 10 years ago. This past September I got the devastating news that my dear friend had taken his own life. I have not been the same since.

"He was kind, loving, funny, compassionate, loyal, honest, and the best person I personally have ever known. He was my friend and I am hurting deeply. I wish he had asked for help. I wish that The Code Green Campaign had been taught to us in paramedic school. That its ok for a hero to ask for help. I hate that its frowned upon that we as paramedics, firefighters, EMTs aren't allowed to ask for help. Having this website has been a blessing that showed up when I needed it most. I miss my great friend."

Anonymous Paramedic

****

In many localities, our first responder applicants are initially screened in regard to their mental stability. Unfortunately, following employment there is often minimal concern for their mental well-being. The authors of the following study discuss a proposed psychological profile of first responders as a collective group.

They note that: ". . . first responders view themselves as having to be strong for others. Showing emotion is considered a type of weakness. This often develops into a hesitancy to seek help, which can lead to worsening mental health. This creates a domino effect. The first responder needs to be psychologically and physically healthy enough to assist others. However, if their own physical and psychological health is ignored, the person in need may not be taken care of either." (Vernberg et al., 2008)

Turning full circle, I'll now utilize tracking data to inquire into the after-effects that 9/11 had on those first responders who served to assist others during and after the incident including their vulnerability to psychological and physical stress consequences.

I'll reference PTSD statistics found within this group from the authors of the following article who noted that: "Responding to critical incidents may result in 5.9-22% of first responders developing psychological trauma and posttraumatic stress disorder. These impacts may be physical, mental, and/or behavioral. This population remains at risk, given the daily occurrence of critical incidents. . ." (Flannery, 2015)

****

"15.136: The hardest calls for me to run these days are the ones involving domestic violence. None of my coworkers know my secret, I was a victim of domestic violence. I will admit, there were times before my volatile relationship, I would think to myself "why do you call when you are just going to go back". I couldn't call because the I lived in the area I worked.

"The shame and guilt of my coworkers, including the police officers, was paralyzing. After becoming the victim (which I still have a hard time accepting, you know because I went back several times... so how am I victim) we need not worry about why they stayed or why I stayed.

"The dynamics of domestic violence are so complex and different for each person, I truly believe it is one of those times you can't understand until you have experienced it for yourself. So I plead to you, don't ever question why someone stays, your very partner may be one who has stayed and hearing those words come from your mouth only cuts deeper in the wound.

"1 in 4 women will be victims of domestic violence. My safe place was my rig with my partner, so please don't take away our safe place with your irrelevant questions as to why someone stayed."

Written by Christina, Paramedic
11 years in EMS

****

I end this chapter with a brief discussion of the impact that being a first responder has on family life. For many years, I took a structured systems family approach looking at the 'identified patient' (IP) within the context of the family system.

I would take into context multi-generational influence or, peer influence coming from outside of the family. For example, which grandparent might be undermining the authority of the parent by being in alliance with the IP (identified patient)?

Were the boundaries between generations rigidified or non-existent? Was one of the parents in alliance with the IP with the other parent pushed out to the fringe within the context of the triangle?

The only way to determine the critical aspects of the prior variables was to observe the system in action. That type of data doesn't seem to be available within the context of available literature pertaining to the family life of the first responder.

Consequently, we are left with snippets of data. One such piece is provided by the authors of the following 2016 study who explored the issues of being a first responder's spouse through a phenomenological viewpoint.

They report that: "Participants included six spouses of first responders in the Southern United States. Five themes emerged from the data: (a) safety, (b) stress, (c) pride, (c.1) civic-mindedness, (d) identity, and (e) finances. The qualitative results identified significant barriers and stressors that exist within the first responder family system and implications for clinical practice with this population." (Porter & Henriksen, 2016)

Another author focused on the children of first responders particularly when one of the parents or more dealt with trauma often on a daily basis. The author noted that: ". . . New York City public school children (N = 8,236) participated in a study examining mental health problems 6 months after the World Trade Center attack. Results revealed that children with emergency medical technician (EMT) family members had a high prevalence of probable posttraumatic stress disorder (PTSD; 18.9%). Differences in rates of probable PTSD among EMTs' and firefighters' children were explained by demographic characteristics. Where EMTs are drawn from disadvantaged groups, one implication of this study is to target EMT families in any mental health interventions for children of first responders." (C. S. Duarte et al., 2006)

As I do my inquiry, I'm impressed by the lack of material pertaining to the families of those who work in these at-risk professions. Alternatively, I can find a multitude of examples of community fund-raising events for those first responders who died in the line of duty. It seems like the day to day lives of folks who serve in these important occupations are too infrequently a topic of discussion.

Based on the above lack of information, I can only speculate on what support components might be engaged to strengthen family ties rather than undermine them. Let's face it, the first responder is engaged in a profession filled with risks that progressively weaken family ties. An example of things at their worst is provided in the following story.

****

"16.64: It's Easter Day, 2016... Three years since my ex wife "kidnapped" my beautiful kids (all under 10) and then divorced me. . . I knew that it was over when I came home from a horrific day. . . Thankfully after getting chewed out by my boss in what I guess was a debriefing (a common occurrence at the station with "why this and why that?") I had no more calls that day. I couldn't wait to get out and go home. I bought a big dinner for my wife and the three kids and just needed some peace and quiet with hopefully a rare, sympathetic ear from my wife (an ER Nurse). As I told her of the events that day I received back "You don't think that I see tough things at my job?".

"Now I'm not saying that I was perfect in our marriage but I was supporting with 'How was your day dear?' whenever she came home and that I would listen to her stories. I thought that I was supportive by listening. Anyhow the marriage went downhill from there with the BS marriage counseling sessions, and the BS time away from the kids on dates and vacations, and all that other stuff with the BS we are all one big happy family.

"Then we get to Easter 2013 and my wife is going to go visit her parents for the holiday. However, she had quit her job without telling me and then a few months later starts to complain about finances as we are now falling behind. I retort with 'GO BACK TO WORK!!!'. She responds with 'A real man would be able to take care of his wife, children, the house, the bills and the vehicles without his wife having to work.'. She left a day early and we didn't talk. When they were scheduled to return she told me that, 'I'm not coming back'.

"With that Three years of Hell started. After this three year divorce battle (her family is very rich) that continues to this day I'm now a middle aged man, living with my mother in a crappy basement with two rooms set up for my children for visitation. Visitation is a funny word as it feels like the kids get to see their father in jail.

". . . I'm at the point where I'm selling everything of value to get through this. I've tried to talk to friends but none of them can relate as they just don't understand the "public safety" thing.

"Everything that I once had is gone. I used to have my own house prior to marriage, could pay my bills, had a vehicle and was generally happy. Now it's all gone and there is no light. All I can see is the pit that I'm in and how much I hate my whining. I'm alone. I just want no more pain."

anonymous paramedic
23 years in EMS.

****

Summary

9/11/2001 was our wake-up call to the danger and challenges facing us in the twenty-first century. One would also assume that we have also awakened to the vulnerabilities that face our first responders. Unfortunately, this does not appear to be the case. As noted above, I and others refer to this group as being members of a high-risk profession.

One of my all-time favorite movies is "Dune". Duke Leto's son, Paul Atreides, takes the Fremen name, Muad'Dib and emerges as the leader for whom the Fremen have been waiting. For me, the highlight of the movie is Paul's statement: "Father – the sleeper has awakened!"

If you're a sci-fi fan and haven't seen this movie, put it on your must do list. If you don't understand my message, I'm suggesting that we all are in need of a wake-up call regarding what these public servants do assist and protect us and the enormous price they pay for their service.

We are indeed in need of an awakening! Fifteen years after 9/11 our CDC is still unable to ascertain how many of our first responders are taking their own lives by suicide. THIS CAN AND MUST BE FIXED! As they say in elections, numbers matter. Based on the varied statistics I've provided in this chapter; I will render a conservative estimate that 15 to 20% of our first responders are struggling with an active PTSD condition.

I've presented you with meta-analysis data that find our current treatments to be simply inadequate in meeting the needs of those with PTSD. I've proposed that the new 'gold standard' needs be the complete and total absence of insomnia, nightmares and intimacy issues from the lives of these vital personnel.

The topic of remission was discussed, with one meta-study noting a range of "8 to 89%." I trust that you find these figures to be as astounding as I do. I challenge this notion that PTSD symptoms simply disappear, referring to the late onset emergence of PTSD symptoms in our aging veterans.

The term "remitted PTSD" was also discussed. I vigorously challenge this belief, holding the perspective that the individual can and must return to a functional pre-trauma state for the treatment to be deemed a success.

Numerous stories were provided throughout the chapter, partially thanks to the permission of the Code Green Campaign. The pain and hardships that the writers of these stories experienced was striking. If they impacted you in a similar manner, please consider contributing to this noteworthy cause at http://code green-campaign.org/.

Finally, I noted the sparsity of literature on the topic of the family and the first responder. As a former family therapist, I envision the emergence of an extended family support system in first responder departments or divisions where children, spouses, etc., receive mutual support through the 'village' they've created. I further envision the administrators of these services consulting with experts in the field to create an environment suitable for thriving rather than the shriveling of self-esteem.

I'd like to end this chapter by referencing an intriguing article written by Rachel Fischell. ("06_53.1donovan - Propranolol use in the prevention and treatment of ptsd in military veterans forgetting therapy revisited.pdf," 2010) The author notes that:

". . . In this world, an emergency medical technician (EMT) forced to witness a violent mutilation following a severe car accident could forget every detail of what they'd observed and avoid the emotional aftermath. . . Administration of propranolol prior to or immediately following traumatic situations to prevent emotional memory consolidation may ensure that no traumatic experience becomes embedded in the amygdala as a non-conscious emotional memory. . .

". . . Because propranolol works to prevent aspects of memory consolidation via reduction of emotion, moral judgments that might arise during such traumatic situations could be affected, thus compromising the quality of patient care.

"In this paper, I will examine the ethical implications of alteration of memory consolidation through emotional dampening and moreover, the inability to make sound moral judgments as a result. Utilizing the current literature . . . I demonstrate that the disadvantages and potential risks of propranolol administration significantly outweigh the potential benefits, especially for the 80 percent of emergency medical personnel who will not develop PTSD.

"Therefore, treatment with propranolol to prevent emotional memory consolidation in emergency medical personnel is unethical and should be prohibited." ("Compos Mentis: Undergraduate Journal of Cognition and Neuroethics - cmv2i2.pdf," 2014)

Later in my book you will read about a non-invasive treatment I've called RESET Therapy. This intervention utilizes a special sound to accomplish the removal of the emotional components of trauma without losing the actual memory of the event as suggested through the use of propranolol. The effect of this intervention appears to be permanent, with no discomforting or residual side-effects. When provided by properly trained and certified personnel within 24 hours following a traumatic event, the intervention can prevent the emergence of PTSD from occurring in the first place.

Reference List:

06_53.1donovan - Propranolol use in the prevention and treatment of ptsd in military veterans forgetting therapy revisited.pdf. https:// msrc.fsu.edu /system/files/Propranolol%20use%20in%20the %20prevention%20and%20treatment%20of%20 ptsd%20in%20military%20veterans%20forgetti ng%20therapy%20revisited.pdf

0017 Violent deaths among first responders: using north carolina violent death reporting system data to inform injury programs -- Austin et al. 21 (Suppl 1): A6 -- Injury Prevention. http:// injurypreven tion.bmj.com/content /21/Suppl_1/A6.2.abstract

!2013-3rded-advocacyhandbook-interactive.pdf. https:// www.emra.org/uploadedfiles/emra/emra_public

ations/books/!2013-3rded-advocacyhandbook-interactive.pdf

Becoming a First Responder: Job Description & Salary Info. http://learningpath.org/articles /Becoming _a_First_Responder_Job_Description_Salary_In fo.html

Bromet, E. J., Hobbs, M. J., Clouston, S. A. P., Gonzalez, A., Kotov, R., & Luft, B. J. (2016). DSM-IV post-traumatic stress disorder among World Trade Center responders 11–13 years after the disaster of 11 September 2001 (9/11). *Psychological Medicine, 46*(4), 771–783. https://doi.org /10.1017/S003329 1715002184

Compos Mentis: Undergraduate Journal of Cognition and Neuroethics - cmv2i2.pdf. http://cm. cognethic.org/cmv2i2.pdf#page=5

Dohrenwend, B. P., Turner, J. B., Turse, N. A., Lewis-Fernandez, R., & Yager, T. J. (2008). War-Related Post-Traumatic Stress Disorder in Black, Hispanic, and Majority White Vietnam Veterans: The Roles of Exposure and Vulnerability. *Journal of Traumatic Stress, 21*(2), 133–141. https://doi.org /10.1002/jts.20327

Duarte, C. S., Hoven, C. W., Wu, P., Bin, F., Cotel, S., Mandell, D. J., ... Markenson, D. (2006). Posttraumatic stress in children with first responders in their families. *Journal of Traumatic Stress, 19*(2), 301–306. https://doi.org/10.1002/jts.20120

Elman, I., Ariely, D., Mazar, N., Aharon, I., Lasko, N. B., Macklin, M. L., … Pitman, R. K. (2005). Probing reward function in post-traumatic stress disorder with beautiful facial images. *Psychiatry Research*, *135*(3), 179–183. https://doi.org/10.1016/j.psychres.2005.04.002

Flannery, R. B. (2015). Treating psychological trauma in first responders: a multi-modal paradigm. *The Psychiatric Quarterly*, *86*(2), 261–267. https://doi.org/10.1007/s11126-014-9329-z

Hopper, J. W., Pitman, R. K., Su, Z., Heyman, G. M., Lasko, N. B., Macklin, M. L., … Elman, I. (2008). Probing Reward Function in Post traumatic Stress Disorder: Expectancy and Satisfaction with Monetary Gains and Losses. *Journal of Psychiatric Research*, *42*(10), 802–807. https://doi.org/10.1016/j.jpsychires.2007.10.008

Huffman, J. C., Niazi, S. K., Rundell, J. R., Sharpe, M., & Katon, W. J. (2014). Essential articles on collaborative care models for the treatment of psychiatric disorders in medical settings: a publication by the academy of psychosomatic medicine research and evidence-based practice committee. *Psychosomatics*, *55*(2), 109–122. https://doi. org/10.1016/j .psym.2013.09.002

Lower Manhattan. (2016, September 6). In *Wikipedia*. https://en.wikipedia.org/w/ index.php?title= Lower_Manhattan&oldid=738060737

Porter, K. L., & Henriksen, R. C. (2016). The Phenomenological Experience of First

Responder Spouses. *The Family Journal, 24*(1), 44–51. https://doi.org/10.1177/ 1066480715 615651

Regehr, C., Hill, J., & Glancy, G. D. (2000). Individual predictors of traumatic reactions in firefighters. *The Journal of Nervous and Mental Disease, 188*(6), 333–339.

Rosen, R. L., Levy-Carrick, N., Reibman, J., Xu, N., Shao, Y., Liu, M., ... Galatzer-Levy, I. R. (2017). Elevated C-reactive protein and posttraumatic stress pathology among survivors of the 9/11 World Trade Center attacks. *Journal of Psychiatric Research, 89*, 14–21. https://doi.org/10.1016/j.jpsychires.2017.01.007

Stanley, I. H., Hom, M. A., & Joiner, T. E. (2016). A systematic review of suicidal thoughts and behaviors among police officers, fire-fighters, EMTs, and paramedics. *Clinical Psychology Review, 44*, 25–44. https://doi.org/10.1016/j.cpr.2015.12.002

Vernberg, E. M., Steinberg, A. M., Jacobs, A. K., Brymer, M. J., Watson, P. J., Osofsky, J. D., ... Ruzek, J. I. (2008). Innovations in disaster mental health: Psychological first aid. *Professional Psychology: Research and Practice, 39*(4), 381–388. https://doi.org/10.1037/a0012663

Veteran IRC firefighter commits suicide shortly after PTSD post on Facebook | Photos. http://www.tcpalm.com/story/news/local/indian-river-county/2016/10/16/indian-river-firefighter/92198338/

Walker, A., McKune, A., Ferguson, S., Pyne, D. B., & Rattray, B. (2016). Chronic occupational exposures can influence the rate of PTSD and depressive disorders in first responders and military personnel. *Extreme Physiology & Medicine, 5*, 8. https://doi.org/10.1186 /s13728-016-0049-x

Watts, B. V., Schnurr, P. P., Mayo, L., Young-Xu, Y., Weeks, W. B., & Friedman, M. J. (2013). Meta-analysis of the efficacy of treatments for posttraumatic stress disorder. *The Journal of Clinical Psychiatry, 74*(6), e541-550. https://doi.org/10.4088 /JCP.12r08225

Chapter Two

Policing

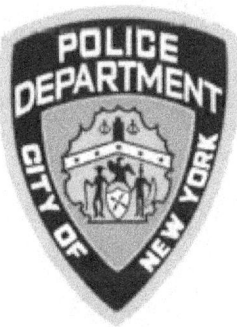

"Law enforcement officers are never 'off duty.' They are dedicated public servants who are sworn to protect public safety at any time and place that the peace is threatened. They need all the help that they can get."

– *Barbara Boxer*

I will be providing you with a developmental history of the law enforcement profession in the U.S. This will include a brief description of personnel employed in police and sheriff's departments as well as a current occupational profile. It is my perspective that law enforcement personnel experience the effects of trauma in a manner that is similar to those of our combat veterans. The difference is that they don't rotate home for 'rest and relaxation.'

As part of each chapter, I will be discussing the rhythm of the job. As an example, a beat may involve a quickened pace within the work day and a shift to a slower or alternative pace when off-duty. Finally, I will recommend how we might go about changing the existing system in preparation for the next emerging era in policing.

A 1989 publication by the National Institute of Justice, U.S. Department of Justice, and the Program in Criminal Justice Policy and Management, John F. Kennedy School of Government, Harvard University, provided a comprehensive overview of the emergence of the current organizational structure of police departments. The contributors refer to three eras of development: the political, reform and community problem-solving eras. The understanding made was that the shift from one era to the next emerged gradually rather than distinctly. Within the 'political era':

". . . American police derived both their authorization and resources from local political leaders, often ward politicians. . . The relationship was often reciprocal: political machines recruited and maintained police in office and on the beat, while police helped ward political leaders maintain their political offices by encouraging citizens to vote for certain candidates, discouraging them from voting for others, and, at times, by assisting in rigging elections.

". . . In the late 19th century, municipal police departments ran soup lines; provided temporary lodging for newly arrived immigrant workers in station houses and assisted ward leaders in finding work for immigrants, both in police and other forms of work. . . Police officers often were recruited from the same ethnic stock as the dominant political groups in the localities and continued to live in the neighborhoods they patrolled.

". . . Control over police by local politicians, conflict between urban reformers and local ward leaders "over the enforcement of laws regulating the morality of urban migrants, and abuses (corruption, for example) that resulted from the intimacy between police and political leaders and citizens produced a continuous struggle for control over police during the late 19th and early 20th centuries." ("The Evolving Strategy of Policing - 114213.pdf," 1988)

"The emergence of the second era was based on the model provided by J. Edgar Hoover's efforts to characterize his FBI agents as upstanding moral crusaders. The authors note that:

"By committing the organization to attacks on crimes such as kidnapping, bank robbery, and espionage-crimes that attracted wide publicity and required technical sophistication, doggedness, and a national jurisdiction to solve, Hoover established the organization's reputation for professional competence and power.

". . . Hoover was also able to maintain an unparalleled record of integrity. That, too, fitted the image of a dogged, incorruptible crime-fighting organization. Finally, lest anyone fail to notice the important developments within the Bureau, Hoover developed impressive public relations programs that presented the FBI and its agents in the most favorable light.

"Struggling as they were with reputations for corruption, brutality, unfairness, and downright incompetence, municipal police reformers found Hoover's path a compelling one. . . Police reformers . . . moved to end the close ties between local political leaders and police. In some states, control over police was usurped by state government. Civil service eliminated patronage and ward influences in hiring and firing police officers.

". . . Professional and bureaucratic authority, especially that which tends to isolate police and insulate them from neighborhood influences, is lessened as citizens contribute more to definitions of problems and identification of solutions." ("The Evolving Strategy of Policing - 114213.pdf," 1988)

****

". . . In squad rooms full of cops, Brian would compare blood pressure meds with his colleagues. Most, if not all, of the police he knew with more than 10 years of service were dealing some kind of medical or psychological issue. At night, Brian would hide his drinking from his wife. He went from sipping whiskey, to downing cheap 100-proof vodka.

"'You see nothing but bodies, I swear, dead people,' he said. 'Car accidents, hangings, suicides, murders, SIDS deaths.' . . . 'I was so angry at this one woman for dying, that I yelled at her,' he said. 'I just didn't want to see another dead body...I should have recognized at that point, it's time for me to back up.'" (Hayasaki, 2014)

****

"The 2012 Bureau of Justice Statistics' Census of State and Local Law Enforcement Agencies (CSLLEA), found there were around 18,000 state and local law enforcement agencies employing at least one full-time officer or the equivalent in part-time officers. As of 2008, more than 1.1 million persons were employed on a full-time basis, including about 765,000 sworn personnel." ("Law enforcement in the United States," 2016)

We will now look at the job description for the occupation of police or sheriff deputy as portrayed in the following occupational profile:

". . . Police officers may work a regular five day, 40-hour week or a compressed work week with 10 or 12 hour shifts. Weekend, holiday and night shifts usually are required because police protection must be provided around the clock. Officers work both indoors and outdoors in all kinds of weather and may be required to stand or walk for hours at a time, or ride in a vehicle for a complete shift." ("Browse Occupations - ALIS OCCinfo: Occupations and Educational Programs," updated 2017)

In regard to shift work, an older study of U.S. Air Force security police (1986) found that:

"[N]ight and rotating shift workers reported significantly more work-related sleep problems than their day shift counterparts. Possibly related to the above conclusion, the perceived level of job effectiveness was significantly lower in night shift workers than day shift workers. Many day shift workers, however, reported that late night activities interfered with their job performance.

"Further, a significant number of night shift workers reported difficulty staying awake on the midnight shift. Clearly, however, the majority of these personnel believed they were more effective working a permanent as compared with a rotating shift schedule." ("Effects of Shift Work on Air Force Security Police Personnel. | National Technical Reports Library - NTIS," 1986)

A recent study referred to the effect that police work has on marital and family difficulties. They suggest that:

". . . many factors add stress to police officers' marriages, including shift work, long hours and unconventional schedules, divided commitment between work and family roles, and perceived personality changes among officers. When police officers carry work-related stress and behaviors into the home, they may experience difficulties in their family relationships. Unfortunately, relatively few researchers have investigated the impact of police work on spouses.

"In this study, we administered a needs assessment to police officers and their spouses to determine the types of difficulties evident in their marriages. Results indicated that officers and spouses generally agreed on stressors and sources of support. Although spouses reported feeling pride about being married to an officer, they also noted financial concerns, work–family conflict, and law enforcement-specific stressors, such as negative public attitudes toward police. Officers and spouses reported relying on friends and family for support more than on professional sources." (Karaffa et al., 2014)

****

"I want to talk about anxiety that seemed to pop up out of nowhere, followed by the persistent dreams and nightmares of a service weapon not firing when needed. This all started happening with about three years on the job, increasing as the years passed into depression, sleeplessness nights, or the ever-present nightmares. I sought help for the depression through department psychologists, and the prescribed pain medication seemed to take the edge off.

"The psychologists were another matter, as repeating my experiences over and over was a waste of time. I was also not going to confide in any of my partners that I felt like I was losing my mind.

"Of course, I had heard of the stress cases, the rubber gun squad and the sick, lame and lazy comments that were part of conversation. I certainly didn't want to be labeled that so I soldiered on." (Steve, 2014)

****

Continuing with the theme of era-to-era change, we are entering the brink of another era in the evolution of policing. As we are all aware, increasing levels of discord is occurring in minority communities. The author of the following article suggests that:

"Police agencies in the U.S. are currently facing a major legitimacy crisis resulting from a spate of high-profile use of force incidents, many involving minority citizens. Recent headlines emphasize that there is now a 'war on cops' and that police officers are facing increasing levels of hostility and violence fueled by a growing anti-police sentiment." (Maguire, Nix, & Campbell, 2016)

We have also become aware of the increasing use of body cameras to capture and document incidents involving officers, in an attempt to diminish allegations of wrongdoing against the police. The following article makes a case that this use is having an opposite effect.

The author suggests that: ". . . Body-worn videos (BWVs) have been proposed as a new way of reducing police use of force, as well as assaults against officers. To date, only a handful of peer-reviewed randomized trials have looked at the effectiveness of BWVs, primarily focusing on use of force and complaints. We sought to replicate these studies, adding assaults against police officers as an additional outcome.

"Using a prospective meta-analysis of multi-site . . . we assess the effect of BWVs on the rates of (i) police use of force and (ii) assaults against officers. Averaged over 10 trials, BWVs had no effect on police use of force . . . but led to an increased rate of assaults against officers wearing cameras. " (Ariel et al., 2016)

A 2015 Gallup annual survey revealed an alarming fact: "American confidence in police has reached a 22-year low. In 2015, only 52% of Americans expressed 'a great deal' or 'quite a lot' of confidence in the police, tying with confidence levels reported in 1993, shortly after LA police officers brutally beat Rodney King. The most troubling part of the national average, however, isn't evident until that statistic is broken down by race. Not only are Americans in general losing confidence in the police, but Black and White Americans have shown starkly different confidence levels for decades." (Initiative, 2015)

****

. . . The majority of my service was either investigating or supervising homicides or death investigations, which number well over 1500. I am now in my 3rd marriage (25 yrs) and have consumed my share of alcohol, which I have now have severely curtailed. I still have nightmares about some of the murder scenes, although they are less frequent. However, certain things still trigger flashbacks, and although I can deal with them, it is hard to relate to my wife what I am going through.

Case in point, tonight, her family planned a family outing at a local restaurant and when we arrived, we were told they could not accommodate our large crowd. The person who organized the outing then suggested that we go to another restaurant, which was the scene of a brutal murder that I worked quite a few years ago. I then told my wife and sister-in-law that I could not go there because it would give me flashbacks. My wife responded by saying you need to 'get over it.'" ("The Police PTSD Paradox | Cops Alive | Police Wellness and Resilience to Stress - Career Survival," 2011)

****

I propose that based on the prior articles and anecdotes, we are experiencing a trend in the public's declining support of law enforcement entities. Consequently, it is time for another era to emerge in the law enforcement community. For lack of a better label, I'll name it the community-based, intra-officer balanced approach.

This approach seeks to sustain the skills, commitment and existing connections to the community of those who serve it over the course of their careers. Simultaneously, it seeks to provide a support system designed to preserve the self-integrity, mental and physical wellness and family integrity of each individual member of the law enforcement profession.

In order to shift to this next phase in policing, we must take a candid look at: the individuals servicing the system; the effects that prolonged stress has on their functioning; the efficacy that current treatment has on remediating their unresolved emotional difficulties; the potential support for change available within their peer community and their administrative systems. I will address each aspect of this approach in the remainder of this chapter.

We begin with the individuals serving in the system. Initially, the police applicant is usually thoroughly vetted and screened. The intent is to select only the mentally healthy candidate to ensure balance and continuity of service to the agency and community.

Then there is the tempo of the occupation. A typical day or shift in law enforcement begins and ends with bookends referred to as standardized routines. This includes a briefing that involves: critical incidents that occurred in the last 24 hours; notifications; missing person reports, etc. After this routine is completed, the onset of uncertainty begins. The following example is provided to illustrate what may occur on a typical day:

****

"You have to strike a balance in the midst of the chaos somewhere, . . . at some point you have to stop and work on reports. This kills you, because your brothers and sisters in arms are getting in fights and scaring up foot pursuits. . . If you get your guy but write a craptastic report, there's a chance he'll slide in court, which defeats the purpose.

". . . Sometimes you find yourself five and six reports behind, so you'd better have taken awesome notes - because as memorable as that first call seemed to be at the time, five calls later you'll have trouble remembering what the basic complaint was, much less names, addresses, relationships, statements, elements of the crime, and so on.

"It's all a mix. There's the boredom of a slow shift spent checking back lots, the adrenaline of a foot pursuit and subsequent street fight, the fear of knowing there are three suspects beating a victim and your backup is blocks away, the headache-afflicted righteous fatigue of processing a DWI.

"After doing all of that, then writing about it in a manner that somehow perfectly describes obscene things in a non-obscene way, you return to the station to your second bookend: refueling the car, unloading it into your POV (personally owned vehicle), and digesting your shift with your squad mates."

("What's it like to be a cop? What happens in your daily life from waking up to going home? - Quora," 2011)

****

What then is it about the 'routine' and uncertainty that changes some of these highly committed, mentally sound public servants into alcohol abusing, physically compromised, personally troubled, burnt out employees? A 2003 revised article provides a dynamic perspective of what likely occurs to the psyche of some of our initially enthusiastic law enforcement officers.

The author notes that: "Policing is an occupation in which, with the passage of time, incident by incident, most officers become conditioned to be less and less familiar with their personal feelings. It is an occupation which promotes a process of emotional insulation or callousness, until officers finally lose touch with the affective or emotional side of their selves. I refer to this process as Systematic Dehumanization.

". . . Insulation is not all bad, it is useful when a person is being overwhelmed by feelings. However, it is a paradoxical defense mechanism. In the short run, it prevents the overwhelming experience of emotional pain, but over the long haul, it begins to prevent the experience of most feelings. . . To make things worse, officers who have been out of touch with their feelings typically feel doubly vulnerable. . . Eventually the officer is cut off from family, friends, and self." ("Peer Assistance Training - Trauma Police Officers are Victims.pdf," ND 2003)

The dangers present in this occupation cannot be understated. One of the most dreaded calls an officer is asked to respond to is one that involves domestic violence, also called intimate partner violence (IPV). A Federal Bureau of Investigation's annual report (2013) was entitled: 'Law Enforcement Officers (LEO) Killed and Assaulted'. Potential cases were confirmed if the narrative included the term 'domestic disturbance' or a domestic disturbance situation was described.

The authors reported the following specifics related to officer fatalities: "116 LEOs were killed while responding to domestic disturbance calls. Ninety-five per cent of these homicides were committed with a firearm. Sixty-seven per cent of LEOs were wearing body armor when killed; however, 52% received the fatal wound to the head/neck.

"Sixty-one per cent of suspects had a criminal history mentioned within the narratives and perpetrators of intimate partner violence (IPV) were more likely to be killed by LEOs than suspects involved in other forms of domestic violence.

"Victims of the domestic disturbance were killed in 21% of the IPV-related LEO homicide cases as opposed to only 5% of other domestic disturbance calls. A firearm was the most common weapon used in the murder of a domestic disturbance victim." (86%)." (Kercher, Swedler, Pollack, & Webster, 2013)

In *Police: The Law Enforcement Magazine*, a featured article is entitled: "Fatal Errors: Surviving Domestic Violence Calls". The authors note that: "Veteran cops have always known that responding to a domestic altercation or assault is a high-risk assignment. The reasons for the danger are plentiful. One or both parties may be intoxicated. Weapons may be involved. Allies to the involved parties may try to intervene, with the officer caught in the middle.

"...The best way to avoid becoming a victim yourself is to remain supremely alert to everything going on around you at the scene of a domestic crime. To stay safe, you will need to control the environment. Freeze the scene to the extent feasible. Do not allow those present to wander in and out of your sight, such as into an adjacent room. If you do, somebody may return with something in hand that means bad news for you. Cops have died in just that way.

"Try to have agitated people sit down. Separate victim and suspect beyond each other's sight. Attempt to persuade uninvolved others to leave the premises, assuming you do not need them as witnesses. Be sure your cover (and you should always have a cover on a domestic call) is watching out for you, too. Work as a team so that you can watch each other's back at all times. Control is the key here. Survival mandates that you keep it on your side." ("Fatal Errors," 2005)

****

". . . I have been out of police work for 7 years. A month after leaving police work I had my first panic attack. I drove myself to the local first aid crew and beat on the doors begging for help. My chest hurt my arms and hands were numb. I thought I was having a heart attack. Went to the doctor who told me my body was use to dealing with a high level of stress and now it doesn't have to it is trying to adjust. He said it could take awhile.

"This is year seven and I'm still having them. Driving and just going out is very taxing. I tried to talk with my family but nobody gets it. I know something is wrong just don't know where to turn. Everybody listens but I have no solutions." ("The Police

PTSD Paradox | Cops Alive | Police Wellness and Resilience to Stress - Career Survival," 2011)

****

Another meaningful article explored an effect that the job has on the physical status of the police officer. New York University at Buffalo researchers now are carrying out one of the first large-scale studies that is investigating the relationship between policing and the emergence of heart difficulties.

". . . Results from Violanti's pilot studies have shown, among other findings, that officers over age 40 had a higher 10-year risk of a coronary event compared to average national standards; 72 percent of female officers and 43 percent of male officers, had higher-than-recommended cholesterol levels; and police officers as a group had higher-than-average pulse rates and diastolic blood pressure." ("Impact Of Stress On Police Officers' Physical And Mental Health -- ScienceDaily," 2008)

Let's also take a look at the correlation between PTSD symptoms reported and the number of traumas experienced by the officers. The suggestion implied in the following study is that those law enforcement personnel with longevity who remain active in policing are more likely to report a corresponding increase in their symptomology. The authors of the following study apparently found this to be the case:

". . . examined 967 diagnostic files of police officers seeking treatment for PTSD. Six hundred twelve (63%) of the referred police officers were diagnosed with PTSD (n = 560) or partial PTSD (n = 52). Police officers reported on average 19.5 different types of traumatic events (range 1-43).

"Those who experienced a greater variety of traumatic events suffered from more PTSD symptoms. Also, women reported more often direct life-threatening or private events as their index trauma than men and suffered from more PTSD symptoms than their male colleagues." (van der Meer et al., 2016)

The effects of fatigue partially produced by overtime demands can play havoc with an officer's life. The authors of the following article have reported that: "The data revealed significant levels of fatigue among officers who reported that they routinely worked more consecutive hours than would be legal in other public service industries. In fact, from the objective measures, levels of fatigue six times higher than those found among shift workers in industrial and mining jobs were discovered.

"In addition, high levels of sleep pathologies were found from the self-report measures of sleep quality where only 26 percent of officers reported averaging the seven or more hours of sleep per day that research finds are minimally required for good health." ("Evaluating the Effects of Fatigue on Police Patrol Officers: Final Report - 184188.pdf," 2000)

Furthermore, when sleep disturbance becomes an ongoing phenomenon, changes in memory and cognitive ability alters. Translated, this means that the affected officer is no longer performing at peak performance levels.

The following 2015 study authors focused on alteration in brain anatomy suggesting that: ". . . there is general consensus that sleep benefits neuronal plasticity, which ultimately supports brain function and cognition. In agreement with this are numerous studies showing that sleep deprivation (SD) results in learning and memory impairments. . .

"Although the molecular mechanisms underlying sleep and memory formation remain to be investigated, available evidence suggests that SD may impair hippocampal neuronal plasticity and memory processes. . .

"When restricted sleep becomes a chronic condition . . . by impairing hippocampal plasticity and function, chronically restricted and disrupted sleep contributes to cognitive disorders and psychiatric diseases." (Kreutzmann, Havekes, Abel, & Meerlo, 2015)

****

"From a police staff psychologist: I still often find young officers who, according to me, have many symptoms of PTSD, refusing to engage in the process. Despite my best effort at encouraging them to seek help, to make a claim, despite the repeated calls of TST members, the officers refuse to make a claim and be properly diagnosed and treated, for fear of repercussion on their career if anybody ever found out.

"Despite the reassurance of the information shared with these officers of the confidential nature of any information received by the Career Development Bureau, the fear persists, and year after year they refuse to seek help. They are left with three options, pay out of pocket for an assessment with a competent and certified mental health practitioner, ask their medical doctor for a referral at a center for such disorders . . . or suffer in silence. Many still take the last option." ("line-of-duty.pdf," 2012)

****

It is my perspective that another option is available but still remains relatively unknown. This option is referred to as rapid remediation accomplished through altering the flight, flight, freeze response in the afflicted individual. A diagnosis is not required for this to happen. It can be accomplished on demand without repercussions to the career path of the individual officer. It can sustain the efficiency and effectiveness of the organization as a whole. I call this intervention RESET Therapy. This solution will be discussed throughout this book.

We now shift to the type of support the law enforcement officer might expect from his/her peers. The police subculture is the focus of the following author's research. He states: "Incorporated in the police subculture is the 'blue wall' or 'code of silence'. This may further motivate officers to be loyal to the organization and forgo disclosure of underlying problems within police organizations. It is estimated that per every suicide, another one thousand officers continue to suffer with PTSD in silence." ("line-of-duty.pdf," 2012)

In addition to self-destructive tendencies, I would be remiss not to also discuss the occasional presence of domestic violence among law enforcement personnel. The author of a 2009 graduate thesis explored the presence of domestic violence within law enforcement families.

The author of this article reported that: "This study included three of the most common aspects of the traditional police sub-culture—burnout, authoritarianism, and cynicism—in order to build and expand upon the previous research and gain a better understanding of the factors that lead police officers to engage in domestic violence.

". . . The results showed that two of the aspects . . . burnout and authoritarianism, were significantly related to psychological domestic violence. As both burnout and authoritarianism increase, the frequency of engaging in psychological domestic violence increases." ("Domestic violence within law enforcement families: The link between traditional police subculture and domestic violence among police - viewcontent.cgi," 2009)

The earlier reference to those who 'suffer in silence' is startling. Because of the seriousness of the prior discussion, it is imperative that we explore this matter further.

****

"We don't know all of the details, all of the gruesome events that haunted his psyche or why he felt that life was simply no longer worth living. We do know that in the summer of 2011, after being exposed to a series of traumatic incidents in the line of duty, including the drowning death of a retired municipal police officer, a suicide and the death of a young child, Sergeant Marshall could no longer function. He was agitated, frustrated and could not organize his thoughts.

"In October 2011, he was hospitalized, plagued by flashbacks from his past of near death experiences and horrific encounters suffered on the job. After being diagnosed with PTSD and receiving treatment in December 2011, he was back at work by mid-January, 2012. His service weapon was returned two weeks later. Then, on April 10th, while at the Southern Georgian Bay Detachment, Sergeant Marshall took his weapon and turned it on himself. He died of a gunshot wound to the head." ("line-of-duty.pdf," 2012)

****

I now discuss the peer-sanctioned use of alcohol within the police subculture. From my perspective, this is the only acceptable outlet that is currently available for the officer to deal with the constant and lingering effects from exposure to trauma. This appears to be further tied into the slowly eroding, psychic poisoning effect of PTSD.

Furthermore, the attitude of peers towards those who experience the effects of emotional trauma is yet another area of concern. One's mindset towards an impaired colleague predicates how an afflicted individual will either reveal and seek help or, repress, avoid and deny developing symptomology.

The following 2016 article suggests that: ". . . little has been written or researched regarding police officers' attitudes to colleagues with mental health issues. Within policing there is a culture that makes it difficult to discuss psychological injury and mental health with colleagues and managers. To do so is often seen as career destroying.

"The inherent cynicism associated with policing, lack of empathy, and macho culture further impedes discussion and ultimately access to support services. Austerity has reduced police training. Inadequate training results in officers not understanding mental health issues. There is an argument that personnel policies and systems victimizes officers and fails to understand their needs." (Bell & Eski, 2016)

****

". . . Since my husband's death on March 8, 1995, I've tried to piece together what made it happen and why. He was the strongest man I've ever known, the rock of our family; our boys idolized him; and now he's gone. He received numerous outstanding evaluations and letters of commendation from numerous national security agencies; he was a foreign counter-intelligence agent. FBI Director Freeh even presented him with a meritorious award posthumously and wrote a tribute about his contributions; he spoke about Bruce's commitment to country at his memorial service. He called him a true American hero. Yet Bruce did not feel fit to live. This proud, brave man died in his boxer shorts, unable even to get dressed. Something is seriously wrong to reduce a man to this." ("» PTSD," n.d.)

****

One might imagine naively that an officer with a solid religious foundation would be more resistant to addictive disorders. Apparently, this is not the case as found by the following 2016 researchers.

"With one exception, the results do not support the notion that enhanced spirituality is associated with lower illness symptoms or perceived stress. Rather, opposing findings were demonstrated involving positive associations between spiritual growth and distress." (Chopko, Facemire, Palmieri, & Schwartz, 2016)

An earlier study (2012) provides similar conclusions. Apparently, a religious belief system is unable to protect the afflicted officer against the cumulative effect of exposure to frequent trauma.

The authors noted that: "This paper evaluates the ability of religion to mitigate the harmful consequences of critical stress using data obtained from a survey of metropolitan police officers ($n = 811$). Contrary to our expectations, we found less religious officer used more adaptive coping strategies when confronted by critical stress incidents than their more religious counterparts." (Clark-Miller & Brady, 2012)

I'll end this particular discussion with a famous quote from Dale Carnegie, American writer, lecturer and the developer of famous courses in self-improvement, salesmanship, corporate training, public speaking, and interpersonal skills. He tells us that: "When dealing with people, remember you are not dealing with creatures of logic, but creatures of emotion."

****

"PHOENIX (CBS5) - Craig Tiger patrolled the streets of Phoenix for 12 years with an unblemished record. But that all changed on a hot summer afternoon in June 2012. He and his partner responded to an emergency call at a north Phoenix park of a man acting wild and threatening people with a bat, including a 4-year-old. 'We gave him numerous verbal commands to drop the baseball bat. He didn't comply. I actually back stepped a couple of times trying to give him even more of an opportunity to drop the baseball bat. He did not,' Tiger said. Both Tiger and his partner fired three shots at the suspect simultaneously. The suspect died at the scene.

"I went home that night to an empty house. It started immediately. I proceeded to self-medicate with alcohol and it started that night. That very night," Tiger said . . . ("Shedding light on PTSD and police - CBS 5 - KPHO," 2014)

****

If the law enforcement officer cannot turn to his faith to protect his inner sense of integrity, what or who can he or she turn to? One would think that his or her peers would be the next option readily available. Unfortunately, the literature suggests that when PTSD emerges, the officer cannot automatically turn to peers because of the macho creed within the subculture. The authors of the following 2016 study explored the subjective impact of trauma, particularly when it led to retirement from active service due to a diagnosis of PTSD.

". . . Chronic exposure to policing trauma was experienced as a domino effect slowly diminishing self-worth and consequently corroding their earlier sense of purpose as police personnel. . . These participants attributed 'felt' distress as directly attributable to organizational factors that left them feeling invalidated, betrayed, and without support." (McCormack & Riley, 2016)

Another 2016 study focused on traumatic stress reaction symptoms among active law enforcement officers. The authors utilized: "snowball sampling to anonymously identify officers willing to participate without involving their employing agencies in any way; participating officers were asked to forward the study's survey instrument along to other potential participants. This methodology virtually eliminates any concerns on the part of officers that reporting psychological symptoms will lead to negative career ramifications such as work reassignment, employment termination, or stigma from the command structure or colleagues.

"Findings indicate that officers' levels of psychological distress were directly related to the number and variety of critical incidents experienced in the course of their careers and to the strength of certain world assumptions . . . relating to self-controllability and the randomness of the world. . . Those officers that experienced more potentially traumatic events experience the world as a more dangerous place, and perceive less meaning and order in the outcomes of their actions." (Green, 2016)

I've provided ample reference to varied research articles, with many of them quite current. While I will provide an overview of this research in the summary aspect of this chapter, I will use the remainder of the chapter to discuss a proposed model for the community based, intra-person balanced approach.

I'll begin with reference to a study of 11 Israeli police first responders who were interviewed about their experience in managing critical incidents of terrorist attacks. The author conducted in-depth interviews and analysis of provided materials. The author surmises that the officers adopted a protective mindset just prior to engaging in the required intervention. This involved: preparation for the worst possible outcome, placing all feeling in a freeze mode and enacting their response based on a prior training model.

The following account is provided: "Once on site they performed, in a robot-like manner, all operations needed to prevent further casualties and make the site safe for rescue vehicles. Once the dead and the wounded were safely evacuated they engaged in site reconstruction and allowed the public to return to their daily activities. On the way home, they reported feelings of professional pride and sorrow over the dead and tried to defreeze their feelings by engaging in routine activities." (Geiger, 2016a)

Despite emotional numbing that was an integral part of their training, first responders revealed intense awareness and vivid traumatic memories of the scene which they seldom shared with family members or therapists. In this macho subculture, treatment was rarely sought since it would entail stigmatization and the preferred mode of relieving tension with the use of black humor with other team members.

****

"One officer who complained to us recalled that when he sat in front of his staff sergeant' delivering his medical note with shaking hands to support a leave for an operational stress injury, the response he got was, 'Well, we've both seen shit, we've been through shit, suck it up.'" ("line-of-duty.pdf," 2012)

****

"Most importantly, the bond uniting first responders, their feeling of being connected with something greater than themselves and to a calling from above, were found to be essential components in their quest for meaning, coherence and purpose. These components allowed for the transformation of the intense memories of disaster and chaos into a source of resiliency and growth that strengthened their faith in their mission of saving lives." (Geiger, 2016b)

I would be inclined to view the prior report as a possible component of a model through which trauma responders' coping skills can be enhanced. The missing piece is the component that could neutralize the build-up effect that accumulates when trauma is experienced over time.

I propose that we have such a tool as elucidated in my prior books. In this sense, RESET Therapy is the key to maintaining the integrity and self-esteem of law enforcement personnel. Imagine if you will, the following scenario.

Upon employment, the hired police officer meets with designated personnel in the department to 'tune in' a target the employee perceives to be somewhat disturbing. The event is not expressed verbally but rather, used to 'light up' the emotional circuitry of the officer's brain. The volume and frequencies that resonate with the target are recorded for later use.

The employee can later be provided with the neuro-modulation instrument and setting for the device upon request at any time without any recrimination. Should an untoward event occur, the emotional aspect of the event can be blocked from doing damage in the first place. Thus, accumulated damage simply doesn't happen. Let me say that again, PTSD doesn't occur in the first place because the emotional components of the trauma are blocked from being stored in the memory circuitry of the brain.

In addition to the voluntary access to the above described process, when critical incidents take place, the involved law enforcement officer also routinely meets with an appropriately certified professional to deprogram from the potential effects of the trauma experience. If this is accomplished fairly rapidly (within a 24-hour period of time), PTSD will not occur.

Next, a support network is established for the spouse and family to provide a form of extended family assistance. This network is there in good times and bad. It is involved in joyful events such as births, graduations, etc., as well as in sad times such as illness, injury or death.

Administratively, the hierarchy modifies itself to support the officer as well as the network. The administrative goal becomes one of providing an effective, competent and skilled force to the community while sustaining the well-being and integrity of its highly trained and skilled personnel.

Harkening back to older times (the political era) in areas with significant minority populations, the force is reflective of the community it serves. It will actively recruit community members to seek appropriate training leading to employment with the force.

Furthermore, administrative personnel support the neuro-scientifically derived position that PTSD in trauma-experienced law officers alters the neuronal circuitry of the brain. This means that PTSD is no longer stigmatized as a personality flaw or sign of inner weakness. Rather, the resetting of the neural circuitry back to a normative mode maintains the well-being of the individual.

By supporting these proposed practices and perspectives administratively, skills and efficiency in the work force are both protected and maintained. All of this is possible with current technology. As noted, the key aspect of this next phase in effective policing is the use of a 'healing sound' that blocks the storage of trauma from the neuronal memory network of the brain.

Summary

Around 1.1 million law enforcement personnel are currently employed in full time positions in the United States. A job description was provided explaining the duties of the position. Among these responsibilities were descriptors of irregular hours as well as rather constant exposure to danger.

A history of the nature of policing was described within the context of three phases that included the political era, the reform era and the community problem-solving era. Societal changes including loss of confidence in law enforcement personnel, particularly in response to policing minority communities thereby heralding the necessity to progress to yet another era. The preponderance of cited articles related to the long-term effects of stress on police officers reveal rather convincing truths. It appears that the longer an officer serves, the more likely he or she is to accumulate the effects of trauma.

The only readily available socially sanctioned mechanism utilized by too many officers is the use and unfortunate abuse of alcohol. Apparently, it is able to at least temporarily shield against the impact produced by accumulating trauma. A defense mechanism referred to as 'insulation' further complicates matters.

As discussed earlier, insulation is a mental defense mechanism that prevents a person from experiencing the awareness of feelings. This can help in the short term in dealing with trauma incidents. Alternatively, over the long-run, this defense can break down dramatically through emergence of suppressed PTSD symptomology.

The topic of an officer's religious belief system and how this might protect against the development of PTSD was discussed. Unfortunately, the data suggests that those without such a strong belief system are likely to cope better.

Health issues are another area of concern within the law enforcement community. "The risk of a coronary event as well as other aspects of police occupational stress including digestive disorders, cardiovascular disease, alcoholism, domestic violence, post-traumatic stress disorder, depression, and suicide (are ever present)." ("The Impact of Stress and Fatigue on Law Enforcement Officers and Ways to Control It," 2014)

In a similar fashion, the 'Thin Blue Line' concept is based upon the denial of weakness, ridicule of mental infirmities and the 'us against them' philosophy. This leaves little room for empathy and support between colleagues. The same can be said for the extended or abbreviated work schedule that leads to disrupted sleep patterns. Alternatively, being part of a functional, healthy family system does seem to provide some measure of protection. The same can be said for positive peer support.

Reference List:

» PTSD: True Story Police Benevolent Foundation. http://www.pbfi.org/?page_id=726

A War on Cops? The Effects of Ferguson on the Number of U.S. Police Officers Murdered in the Line of Duty - Maguire Nix - Campbell -2016- War on Cops.pdf. file:///C:/Users/ User-PC/Downloads /Maguire%20Nix%20-%20Campbell%20-2016-%20War%20on %20Cops.pdf

Abstracts Database - National Criminal Justice Reference Service. https://www.ncjrs.gov /App/ AbstractDB/AbstractDBDetails.aspx?id=241457

Ariel, B., Sutherland, A., Henstock, D., Young, J., Drover, P., Sykes, J., ... Henderson, R. (2016). Wearing body cameras increases assaults against officers and does not reduce police use of force: Results from a global multi-site experiment. *European Journal of Criminology*, 14773708 16643734. https://doi .org/10.1177/147737081 6643734

Bell, S., & Eski, Y. (2016). "Break a Leg—It"s all in the mind': Police Officers' Attitudes towards

Colleagues with Mental Health Issues. *Policing, 10*(2), 95–101. https://doi. org /10.1093/police /pav041

Browse Occupations - ALIS OCCinfo: Occupations and Educational Programs. https://occinfo.alis .alberta.ca /occinfopreview/info/browse-occupations .html

Chopko, B. A., Facemire, V. C., Palmieri, P. A., & Schwartz, R. C. (2016). Spirituality and health outcomes among police officers: empirical evidence supporting a paradigm shift. *Criminal Justice Studies, 29*(4), 363–377. https://doi.org /10.1080/1478601X .2016.1216412

Clark-Miller, J., & Brady, H. C. (2012). Critical Stress: Police Officer Religiosity and Coping with Critical Stress Incidents. *Journal of Police and Criminal Psychology, 28*(1), 26–34. https://doi. org/10.1007/s11896 -012-9112-8

Domestic violence within law enforcement families: The link between traditional police subculture and domestic violence among police - view content .cgi. http://scholar commons .usf. edu /cgi/view content .cgi?article=2861& context=etd

Effects of Shift Work on Air Force Security Police Personnel. | National Technical Reports Library - NTIS. https://ntrl.ntis.gov/NTRL /dashboard/searchResults/titleDetail/ADA17176 5.xhtml

Evaluating the Effects of Fatigue on Police Patrol Officers: Final Report - 184188.pdf. https:// w ww.ncjrs.gov/pdffiles1/nij/grants/184188 .pdf

Fatal Errors: Surviving Domestic Violence Calls. http://www.policemag.com/channel/patrol/articl es/2005/01/fatal-errors-surviving-domestic - violence-calls.aspx

Geiger, B. (2016). An inside look at Israeli police critical incident first responders. *Contemp orary Social Science*, *0*(0), 1–18. https://doi. org/10.1080 /21582041.2016.1228012

Green, D. (2016). Traumatic Stress, World Assumptions, and Law Enforcement Officers. *All Graduate Works by Year: Dissertations, Theses, and Cap stone Projects*. http://academi cworks.cuny.edu /gc_etds/1387

Hayasaki, E. (2014, March 14). Life of a Police Officer: Medically and Psychologically Ruinous. *The Atlantic*. http://www. theatlantic.com/health /archive/2014/03/life-of-a-police-officer-medically-and-psycho logically-ruinous/284324/

Impact Of Stress On Police Officers' Physical And Mental Health -- ScienceDaily. https://www. sciencedaily.com/releases/2008/09/080926105029.htm

Initiative, P. P One institution, two different views: How Black and White Americans regard the police | Prison Policy Initiative. http://www. Prison policy.org/blog/2015/07/02/police_confidence/?gclid=Cj0KEQjwkdHABRCHiZ2gs6yGh50BEi QAA91Wlnl1YtwcKVSIQ0enpBDy2xydagzum b0s-FS47Ljoe1ka AlYL8P8HAQ

Karaffa, K., Openshaw, L., Koch, J., Clark, H., Harr, C., & Stewart, C. (2014). Perceived Impact of Police Work on Marital Relationships. *The Family Journal*, 1066480714564381. https:// doi.org /10.1177/1066480714564381

Kercher, C., Swedler, D. I., Pollack, K. M., & Webster, D. W. (2013). Homicides of law enforcement officers responding to domestic disturbance calls. *Injury Prevention: Journal of the Inter* national Society for Child and Adolescent Injury Prevention, 19(5), 331–335. https://doi.org /10.1136/injuryprev-2012-040723

Law enforcement in the United States. In *Wikipedia*. https://en.wikipedia.org/w/index.php?title=Law _enforcement_in_the_United_States&oldid=742 582163

line-of-duty.pdf. http://www.cbc.ca/manitoba /features/rcmp-ptsd/images/line-of-duty.pdf

McCormack, L., & Riley, L. (2016). Medical discharge from the "family," moral injury, and a diagnosis of PTSD: Is psychological growth possible in the aftermath of policing trauma? *Traumatology*, 22(1), 19–28. https://doi.org/10.1037 /trm0000 059

Peer Assistance Training - Trauma Police Officers are Victims.pdf. http://policesuicide. spcollege.edu /assets/Trauma%20Police%20Officers%20are% 20Victims.pdf

Police Officer - Occupation Profile - ALIS OCCinfo: Occupations and Educational Programs. http://occinfo.alis.alberta.ca /occinfopreview /info/browse-occupations/ occupation-profile. html?id=71003122

Shedding light on PTSD and police - CBS 5 - KPHO. http://www.cbs5az.com/story /26643380/ shedding-light-on-ptsd-and-police

Steve. (2014, November 14). PTSD progression not recognized by police departments. http:// www.policeptsd.com/2014/11/14/ptsd- progression-not-recognized-by-police- departments/

The Evolving Strategy of Policing - 114213.pdf. http://www.innovations.harvard.edu/sites/default/files/114213.pdf

The Police PTSD Paradox | Cops Alive | Police Wellness and Resilience to Stress - Career Survival. http://www.copsalive.com/the-police-ptsd-paradox/

van der Meer, C. A. I., Bakker, A., Smit, A. S., van Buschbach, S., den Dekker, M., Westerveld, G. J., ... Olff, M. (2016). Gender and Age Differences in Trauma and PTSD Among Dutch Treatment-Seeking Police Officers. *The Journal of Nervous and Mental Disease*. https://doi.org/10.1097/NMD.0000000000000562

What's it like to be a cop? What happens in your daily life from waking up to going home? - Quora. https://www.quora.com/Whats-it-like-to-be-a-cop-What-happens-in-your-daily-life-from-waking-up-to-going-home

Chapter Three

Firefighting

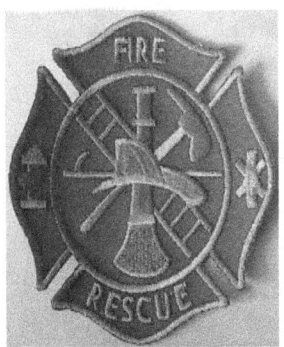

I have no ambition in this world but one, and that is to be a fireman. The position may, in the eyes of some, appear to be a lowly one; but we who know the work which the fireman has to do believe that his is a noble calling. Our proudest moment is to save lives. Under the impulse of such thoughts, the nobility of the occupation thrills us and stimulates us to deeds of daring, even of supreme sacrifice.

Chief Edward F. Croker FDNY Circa 1910

"The history of firefighting in America can be traced . . . to Jamestown, VA, the first permanent English settlement in the New World. Founded in 1607 by colonists from the London Company, Jamestown was under the command of Captain James Smith. It did not take long for fire to begin taking its toll on the new settlers.

"In January 1608, a devastating fire destroyed most of the colonist's provisions and lodgings. Smith made a concise assessment of the situation: 'I begin to think that it is safer for me to dwell in the wild Indian country than in this stockade, where fools accidentally discharge their muskets and others burn down their homes at night.'

". . . The communities that sprang up around three of the best harbors - Boston, New York and Philadelphia - soon faced a number of social problems involving housing, sanitation, water supply and the danger of fire. . . In 1648, New Amsterdam (later New York) Governor Peter Stuyvesant stood firmly on his peg leg and appointed four men to act as fire wardens. They were empowered to inspect all chimneys and to fine any violators of the rules.

"The city burghers later appointed eight prominent citizens to the "Rattle Watch" - these men volunteered to patrol the streets at night carrying large wooden rattles. If a fire was seen, the men spun the rattles, then directed the responding citizens to form bucket brigades.

". . . Most notable among the famous Americans who helped shape the country and the fire service was Benjamin Franklin, a writer, printer, philosopher, scientist, statesman of the American Revolution - and a fireman. . . In 1736, Franklin founded the Union Fire Company in Philadelphia, which became the standard for volunteer fire company organization." ("Firefighting in Colonial America," 2013)

****

"In February 2005, Mack attended a structure fire with his partner. Despite textbook execution on their behalf, his partner fell through the floor to where the fire had started. When he fell, he knocked off Mack's oxygen mask, rendering him semi-unconscious.

"As he came to, his partner was screaming for the hose line to fight the fire, and when they tried to radio in a mayday call the batteries were dead, meaning Mack had to leave his partner in the burning building to get help.

"The two survived with smoke inhalation, but that six-minute window changed Mack's life forever. He said he started exhibiting symptoms of PTSD almost immediately — he was fearful of going back to work, his drinking went through the roof, he wasn't sleeping, lost interest in almost everything, and developed anger issues.

"He said he attended a debriefing session after the incident, and a month after the fire he sought counseling. . . 'My best buddy was my beer bottle — that's all I wanted. That was my comfort, that was my sanity,' he said." ("Post-traumatic stress disorder," 2012)

****

The following report contains statistical information through 2015 regarding the numbers and descriptions of U.S. fire departments and firefighters. "NFPA estimates there were approximately 1,160,450 local firefighters in the U.S. in 2015. Of the total number of firefighters 345,600 (30%) were career firefighters and 814,850 (70%) were volunteer firefighters.

"Most of the career firefighters (71%) worked in communities that protected 25,000 or more people. Most of the volunteer firefighters (95%) were in departments that protected fewer than 25,000 people. Nearly two-thirds (65%) of volunteer firefighters have more than 5 years of service.

"There are an estimated 29,727 fire departments in the U.S. Of these, 2,651 departments were all career, 1,893 were mostly career, 5,421 were mostly volunteer and 19,762 were all volunteer. In the U.S., 13,500 departments provided EMS with basic life support, 4,617 departments provided EMS with advanced life support and 11,610 departments did not provide EMS.

"The main duties of a full-time firefighter are to help protect the public in emergency situations. They respond to a wide variety of calls, such as car crashes, chemical spills, flooding, water rescue and general rescue as well as fires.

"With many fire crews being trained as first responders they can provide first aid until the arrival of ambulance personnel. . . All staff wear uniforms, and 24-hour shift work is a standard requirement of the job. The work can be stressful and dangerous but there is a great deal of job satisfaction to be gained from providing such a valuable service to the community." ("NFPA report - U.S. fire department profile," 2017)

The structure-framework for this chapter will consist of the following components: job tempo, family, cumulative trauma exposure, critical incidents, Critical Incident Stress Debriefing

(CISD), the male prevalent culture, longitudinal health impact, employee burnout, stress effects and their association with PTSD, and suicide.

We begin with a discussion of the tempo/pace of the firefighting profession. The setting is that of a large city (Chicago) containing low-income areas including high rises. This is one of the busiest stations in the city averaging 400 calls a month during the summer months.

The author of the following article reports on the perspective of one of the firefighters who notes that: "'It comes natural now,' says Johnson of the action, the fast pace. `If you think about it, you go crazy. After seeing so many tragic things, you just block it out. . . Here you don`t get any rest. We`re like human bouncing balls.'

". . . the firefighters talk about the importance of ventilation-sawing, tearing or puncturing a roof so that the smoke can escape. The quicker you get through a roof, the easier it`s going to be for firefighters to search for victims and extinguish the flames. It is backbreaking work that must be carried out with precision. . . `The first five minutes of a fire makes it or breaks it. Either we gain control of the fire, or the fire gains control of us.'

". . . You've got to know how to feel your way along the walls while crawling on your belly, because if you lift your head the smoke can choke you. Along the way you will step on nails, hypodermic needles, broken glass, rats. You must sense the heat with your ears because your gloved hands will not feel it. And finally, you must remember how and when to get out.'

"Willie Northern is one of the men assigned to Engine 19. 'The hardest part of the job is seeing death' he says. 'I've seen some babies burnt up real bad. It really hurts when you see those children. And when you find out the circumstances, sometimes you say, 'Why did this happen?'

". . . Just moments before dinner, another call comes in. One long bell sounds for a fire in the 200 block of West 33d Street. The calls for help are transmitted in a dispassionate language of loud monotone alarms that arrive unexpectedly. . . The firefighters grab their gear, climb into their knee-high boots, and climb aboard the truck." ("A Day In The Life Of Chicago's Busiest Firefighters," 1989)

I'll now shift to the role of the family in buffering job related stressors or alternatively, how they may soften the impact of stress for one of their members. Societally, the family is designated to function as a core component, ensuring the continuity of the culture.

Part of this purpose is to assist the afflicted individual to be able to rebound from persistent challenge. When viable, the family is central in addressing trauma and adversity. When weakened or rigidified, the family becomes unable to cope with disruptive transitions or crisis, or for that matter with chronic multi-stress conditions.

A perception exists that divorce among firefighters highly exceeds those of the general public, primarily due to the stressful nature of the job. Results of a study suggest that this may or may not be true. The following writer noted that: "Data was provided by 1,456 firefighters in 31 departments across the country. Our sample had a larger number of firefighters who were in the youngest age bracket (19 to 29 years old) than the general population data that was available.

". . . In our sample, 77 percent of male firefighters were currently married and 11.8 percent were currently divorced. This compared to 57.5 percent married in the U.S. population and 9.4 percent divorced. For female firefighters, the rate of current marriage was 42.6 percent and current divorce was 32.1 percent, compared with 55.4 percent married and 10.4 percent currently divorced in the general population. ("Firefighter divorce," 2015)

The prior report reveals that the male firefighter is more likely to be in a stable family relationship while the female appears to be at risk within the context of a viable marital relationship.

****

"I was a badass firefighter, a seasoned veteran, even looked up to. How could I be seen as weak? Simply put I couldn't, so I pushed on, I drank more, worked more, and everything around me began to crack and fall apart. My inability to seek help had real consequences. My family life was in tatters, my finances were in ruin, my health declined, and my madness grew.

"Finally, on a warm July night, drunk again I crawled into the cab of my pickup truck, closed the garage door, found an appropriately sad song, and passed out with the truck running. Only by chance did my wife discover my suicide attempt; without her intervention my effort would have been a success." ("Firefighter suicide report.pdf," 2012)

****

Fortunately, in the preceding example, a caring family member was able to intervene, thereby averting a potential tragedy. Unfortunately, in many other cases, intervention doesn't occur and trauma ensues. I will discuss suicide later in the chapter but at this point, I focus on the disruption caused by cumulative stress exposure.

Unfortunately, minimal research on cumulative trauma exposure among first responders has been reported. The authors of the following 2016 study provided a series of assessments to a sample of urban firefighters on a yearly basis over the entirety of their careers noting that: ". . . The results of this study predict that as a career in the fire service progresses, as age increases, as the average hours of sleep decrease, as their rank within the department rises, as the number or critical incidents attended, and as the number of critical incident stress debriefings attended increase, all of the mental disorders measures will increase." (Pelham, 2016)

I find the results from this well-developed longitudinal study to have serious implications that pertain to the above listed variables. All of these experiences lead collectively to an increase in psychopathology.

For clarification purposes, a critical incident is: "any event that has a stressful impact sufficient enough to overwhelm the usually effective coping skills of an individual. Critical incidents are abrupt, powerful events that fall outside the range of ordinary human experiences. . . Research has shown that critical incident stress affects up to 87% of all emergency service workers at least once in their careers." ("Critical Incident Stress," 2007)

****

". . . You remember your critical incident call, probably in great detail. It may have been a call that has changed your life and/or values. An officer-involved shooting, a hostage standoff, a mass suicide, an infant at the bottom of the pool, a family trapped in a burning car, a six-year-old versus a semi-truck, the domestic violence call from hell, a school shooting, a rape, a natural disaster, a senseless homicide, the situation that hit too close to home, the déjà vu call--the list is infinite.

"It is important that the definition of a critical incident remain fluid in your mind; what may affect you will not necessarily affect another officer, and vice versa. For example, an officer who has children might be affected by responding to the traumatic death of a child more than an officer who has no children." ("Critical Incident Stress," 2007)

****

I find it necessary to clarify Critical Incident Stress Debriefing (CISD), which is a formalized, structured method whereby a group of rescue and response workers reviews the stressful experience of a disaster. CISD was developed to assist first responders, such as fire and police personnel; it was not meant for the survivors of a disaster or their relatives." ("Types of Debriefing Following Disasters - PTSD," 2007)

A 2016 article about Critical Incident Stress Debriefing takes a rather harsh look at this type of intervention reporting that: "Despite a lack of proof that expressing feelings right away is good, the U.S. has an industry of people, called critical incident stress debriefers, whose job it is to converge on disaster sites and get people to talk about their feelings.

"Not necessarily mental health experts, debriefers sent by city or county health, fire or police departments have had training in what to say to encourage emoting after a disaster. They head to scenes of death and destruction caused by Hurricane Katrina, floods in Iowa or fires throughout California, not to mention human-made horrors like the 9/11 attack on the World Trade Center or the Columbine and Virginia Tech school shootings. Yet a 2006 review of studies on such debriefings in the Review of General

Psychology found, in general, either no benefit or worse outcomes from the interventions.

"'If it's immediately after an upheaval, it's completely foolish to do that,' says James Pennebaker, chair of psychology at the University of Texas at Austin. 'Some people naturally talk and listen to others. If they don't want to talk about it, they don't. If they do, they do. They may need help in two months, but they may not want help then.'" ("Debunking debriefing," 2008)

To address this matter more formally, I turned to the U.S. Department of Veterans Affairs – National Center for PTSD to clarify governmental perspective pertaining to the viability of this intervention. The following material was forthcoming: ". . . [R]ecent research indicates that psychological debriefing is not always an appropriate mental-health intervention. Available evidence shows that, in some instances, it may increase traumatic stress or complicate recovery. Psychological debriefing is also inappropriate for acutely bereaved individuals. . .

"A recent review of eight debriefing studies, all of which met rigorous criteria for being well-controlled, revealed no evidence that debriefing reduces the risk of PTSD, depression, or anxiety; nor were there any reductions in psychiatric symptoms across studies. Additionally, in two studies, one of which included long-term follow-up, some negative effects of CISD-type debriefings were reported relating to PTSD and other trauma-related symptoms.

"Therefore, debriefings as currently employed may be useful for low magnitude stress exposure and symptoms or for emergency care providers. However, the best studies suggest that for individuals with more severe exposure to trauma, and for those who are experiencing more severe reactions such as PTSD, debriefing is ineffective and possibly harmful." ("Types of Debriefing Following Disasters - PTSD," updated 2016)

With the above perspective in mind, I would advise that the prudent fire administrator explore alternative interventions. Of course, I have such an intervention in mind called RESET Therapy.

****

"It's the middle of the night. I'm sitting alone someplace on West Street. My helmet is perched on the back of my head. I'm leaning forward, elbows on my knees, and my face is in my hands. A cigarette burned to the filter is between my fingers. It's dark, and a misting rain is falling. The smell is pretty pungent. Smoke is slowly rising from the piles of steel that used to be the World Trade Center.

"Suddenly, I look up, and Tommy is standing there in front of me. He and Adam are both looking at me emotionless with stone faces. Then they turn and look back toward the wreckage. They slowly raise their arms and point to the middle of 'The Pile.'

They say nothing. They hold that pose for a few moments; then their faces turn back toward mine. Tommy's eyes are very dark, and tears are about to fall onto his cheeks. Adam is standing behind him, about three feet to his left. He just stands there and continues to stare at me with an almost helpless look on his face. Slowly their arms drop back down to their sides ...

".........BANG!!!!!!!!!!!!!!!

"... *"What is wrong with me?"* I slide my feet out of the side of the bed. I am shaking. The sheets are wet, and my sweat is cold. I feel as if somebody just beat me with a cane. . . It's past midnight; I am sitting in bed soaking wet, crying, wondering what is

wrong with me and will it EVER stop."
("Login," 2010)

****

At this point, it's time to discuss the unholy alliance of alcohol, cumulative stress and trauma. Use of alcohol is a common feature shared in the bonding experience among many service personnel. It is part of the culture of masculine organizations. I'll begin with further inquiry into the 'macho man' veneer behind the 'if it doesn't kill you, it makes you stronger' facade.

The authors of the following 2015 study focused on fire stations in a major metropolitan area reporting that: ". . . [T]he emotional cultures of firefighting units were defined by two emotions: joviality and companionate love. In addition, emotion suppression, work-family conflict, risk taking and health problems emerged as central themes." (O'Neill & Rothbard, 2015)."

Another study conducted in 2013 explored components of stigma pertaining to mental illness within a predominately male dominated occupation finding that: ". . . Frequently occurring categories of stigma for first responders were discrimination, disbelief, loss of status, and shame. . . Loss of status was of particular concern for first responders, suggesting that stigma might impact first responders differently from the general population, due in part to the unique characteristics of their profession." ("JMGC-Vol-3-Is-3.pdf," 2013) Because of a number of factors, first responders are generally resistant to counseling intervention. This response set is also found in military personnel and is clearly one component in primarily male dominant organizations. The following research targeted deep-seated and bothersome material leading to burnout:

A 2016 study of French firefighters focused on the contributions of physical exercise, burnout and coping strategies in relation to firefighting-related injuries. The authors collected from a population-based sample of 220 male firefighters. As reported: ". . . the nature and site of the injuries and the relationships among firefighter injuries, physical exercise, burnout and coping strategies were examined. Sprains were the most prevalent type of injury (98%), followed by tendinitis (40%) and muscle tears (30%).

"More than two thirds of these injuries were located at the ankle. Weekly hours of physical exercise, cognitive weariness at work, social support seeking, problem-focused coping and emotional exhaustion were significantly related to these injuries."

(Vaulerin, d'Arripe-Longueville, Emile, & Colson, 2016)

A particular problem found within the first responder community is the difficulty in addressing the occurrence of burnout. Fearing that he or she will be stigmatized by others, they are inclined to suppress this aspect of functioning thereby building up internalized distress. I'll begin this topic with a definition of the phenomena.

The editors of *Psychology Today* have opined that burnout is not a simple result of long hours. Rather, the cynicism, depression and lethargy aspects of burnout are likely to occur because: "Burnout is a state of chronic stress that leads to: physical and emotional exhaustion; cynicism and detachment; feelings of ineffectiveness and lack of accomplishment.

"When in the throes of full-fledged burnout, you are no longer able to function effectively on a personal or professional level. However, burnout doesn't happen suddenly. You don't wake up one morning and all of a sudden 'have burnout.'

"Its nature is much more insidious, creeping up on us over time like a slow leak, which makes it much harder to recognize. Still, our bodies and minds do give us warnings, and if you know what to look for, you can recognize it before it's too late." (Editors, 2016)

So, if you don't notice it, what do you do? A sample of career firefighters involved in a computer-based, self-administered, health assessment survey produced the following results: "The majority of the sample (n = 160) consumed alcohol (89%), with approximately one-third (34%) having a drinking binge in the past 30 days. . . Drinking levels observed in this study exceed those of the general adult population, including college students. Thus, it appears that firefighters represent an at-risk drinking group." (Piazza-Gardner et al., 2014)

In addition to drinking, the prolonged effects of stress with accompanying burnout lead to psychophysiological vulnerability. The next component of this chapter will focus on the most prevalent symptoms of this phenomenon. This will include physical manifestations of prolonged stress in the following order: cardiovascular disease, low back pain, obesity, sleep disorders, and post-traumatic stress disorder.

Because of the seriousness of damage to the cardiovascular system resulting in upwards of 45% of deaths among those firefighters who expire on duty, I shall utilize the following study in regard to clarifying the likely causation for underlying, silently emerging Cardio-Vascular Disease (CVD).

The authors report that: "Recently, our understanding of CVD in the fire service has significantly improved and provides insight into the risks of firefighting (that) relate primarily to the interaction of physically and psychologically stressful duties with underlying CVD. These strenuous duties provoke a physiology of cardiovascular arousal in association with acute firefighting activities, which usually have no long-term consequences in healthy firefighters, but can trigger pathophysiologic changes and acute CVD events in firefighters with underlying heart disease.

". . . Despite the strenuous nature of emergency duty, the prevalence of low fitness, obesity and other CVD risk factors in the fire service are high. Robust evidence for both highly prevalent risk factors and the interaction of strenuous duties with underlying Cardiac fatalities are the leading cause of death among all firefighters." (Sen, Palmieri, & Greenhalgh, 2016)

An earlier study explored cardiovascular events that "account for 45% of deaths among firefighters on duty. In contrast, such events account for 22% of deaths among police officers on duty, 11% of deaths among on-duty emergency medical services workers, and 15% of all deaths that occur on the job." (Kales, Soteriades, Christophi, & Christiani, 2007)

****

"A rookie firefighter helping to battle one of his first major blazes died yesterday afternoon, apparently of a heart attack, minutes after unraveling water hoses during a giant fire at a Staten Island auto repair shop, the authorities said.

". . . Moments after Mr. Gorumba's engine arrived, firefighters began pulling hoses off their truck and began connecting them to hydrants. Mr. Gorumba was assigned to ensure that the hoses, which might contort and spin out of control from intense water pressure, flowed properly.

". . . Mr. Gorumba was the sixth firefighter to die on duty this year and the fourth in 10 months to die of a heart attack on the job. Three firefighters died fighting a blaze at a Queens hardware store in June.

"In January, two firefighters, . . . suffered heart attacks while on duty. Firefighter Franklin died about an hour after a fire at a

Bronx tenement, and Firefighter McLoughlin died while working out on a treadmill while on duty. Firefighter Kenneth Kerr died of a heart attack in November after fighting a Bronx fire." (Jones, 2001)

****

We next review a 2014 Finnish study that includes sleep disturbance within the context of an investigation of the prevalence of low back pain among Finnish firefighters. The authors discussed the results from a prospective study that included 360 actively working firefighters. The participants responded to a questionnaire in 1996, 1999 and 2009. The outcome variables were radiating and local low back pain during the preceding year.

The authors reported that: "During the 13-year follow-up, the prevalence of radiating low back pain increased from 16 to 29% . . . and that of local low back pain from 28 to 40%. . . This is the first prospective study to show that low back symptoms are common and persistent among firefighters and that sleep disturbances strongly predict membership of a radiating pain trajectory. Occupational health and safety personnel, as well as the firefighters themselves, should recognize sleep problems early enough in order to prevent back pain and its development into chronic pain." (Lusa, Miranda, Luukkonen, & Punakallio, 2014)

****

"I was injured in the line of duty as a volunteer fireman at a fully involved house fire 3 years ago this June. A fellow fireman who was on a ladder +/-14 feet above my head, lost his footing and fell headfirst / backwards off the ladder towards a concrete surface and I jumped under him to break his fall as I was footing the ladder for him.

". . . As courageous as that may seem and a hero I may be to some (although not recognized by the Fire Department as it was not considered rescuing someone from inside the fire building and they typically call that a 'Grab,' no pun intended); I would have expected any one of my fellow brothers to do the same for me as that is a fireman's code.

"Unfortunately, not only have I been on Medical leave since the incident, but I feel as though my Fire department, both friends and the Chiefs office have simply forgotten about me altogether.

". . . I am so limited in what I do on a daily basis like climbing a flight of simple stairs to my front door requiring me to use the ramp instead, getting in and out of my car, driving more than 15 miles. . . going to the bathroom, walking more than a block, any physical activity in which my children beg me to play with them and simply cannot . . .

"I am sure many of you have stories that can relate, but I (find) that my mind can not sit still as I feel inadequate as a man, although I have the greatest and most supporting woman, kids and family in my life. It truly is the only thing that keeps me from doing myself in. – Marc." ("Fireman Back Pain,")

****

As an occupational group, firefighters have one of the highest prevalence rates of obesity. The author of the following 2013 article reported that: "Four focus groups were conducted with firefighters of every rank as Phase I of the FORWARD study which was designed to assess health behavioral and occupational characteristics related to obesity in firefighters.

"Analysis revealed five main themes of central importance to firefighters: (1) fire station eating culture; (2) night calls and sleep interruption; (3) supervisor leadership and physical fitness; (4) sedentary work; and (5) age and generational influences. The results showed a strong interrelationship between occupational and health behavioral causes of obesity in firefighters." (Dobson et al., 2013)

The authors of the following article assessed 6,933 firefighters from 66 U.S. fire departments using a validated screening tool noting that: "A total of 37.2% of firefighters screened positive for any sleep disorder (difficulties) including obstructive sleep apnea (OSA), 28.4%; insomnia, 6.0%; shift work disorder, 9.1%; and restless legs syndrome, 3.4%. Compared with those who did not screen positive, firefighters who screened positive for a sleep disorder were more likely to report a motor vehicle crash (adjusted odds. . . and were more likely to self-report falling asleep while driving." (Barger et al., 2015)

The last medically related area to be discussed is the issue of PTSD. According to the National Center for Post-Traumatic Stress Disorder (2012), PTSD is a serious anxiety disorder that can happen following a traumatic experience or witnessing an event. (Beyler, 2001).

****

"There had been a crash involving a child and a vehicle — and Darren, a firefighter . . .

remembers the boy asking him if he was going to die. . . "And then he reached up and actually touched my face, so I'm trying to comfort him but trying not to tell him 'yes' or 'no,' . . . Over the course of the next few weeks, the incident continued to bother Darren — he said he wasn't sleeping well and became more irritable.

". . . Darren said that seeing the counsellor helped, but from time to time he still finds himself thinking about the incident. He has stopped seeing his counsellor, but said he still experiences some anxiety when he attends or hears about calls involving pedestrians and vehicles — something he doesn't think will ever go away.

". . . He said his biggest concern was that if he was constantly being distracted by memories of the incident he would be putting those working with and under him at risk — a chance he wasn't willing to take. 'You can't hesitate — you have a fraction of a second to make a decision that's going to affect someone's life,' Darren explained.

"I had to make sure I was focused on what I was doing and not thinking about this thing.

I didn't want to be responsible for someone else because I wasn't paying attention, I wasn't at the top of my game." ("Post-traumatic stress disorder," 2012)

****

The following study sought to address the role of multiple traumas on other mental health occurrences, such as depression and alcohol misuse, among emergency workers. The researchers targeted the prevalence of post-traumatic stress disorder, depression and alcohol misuse in a sample of current and retired fire-fighters and examine their relationship with cumulative trauma exposure.

They reported that: ". . . Retired fire-fighters reported significantly greater levels of symptomatology, with the prevalence estimates of post-traumatic stress disorder at 18% . . . depression at 18% . . . and heavy drinking at 7%. There was a significant positive linear relationship between the number of fatal incidents attended and rates of post-traumatic stress disorder, depression and heavy drinking." (Harvey et al., 2016)

A final note on this topic is to be found in the following article, wherein the author reports that due to the organizational nature of Fire Departments: "Firefighters and firefighter leaders often relive experiences, responding to structures where deadly fires previously occurred. Reliving deadly experiences are a normal operational function for department leaders. Often departmental protocol requires firefighter leaders to relive dangerous or deadly situation to perfect fire suppression strategies and tactics." (Cunningham, 2002)

We next explore the amassing of failure to cope experiences leading to self-destructive ideation and engagement in actual activity directed towards the ending of life. Those survivors who are left behind begin anew the recycling of trauma in their lives.

****

". . . We called our son Jackie. He took his own life on June 25, 2011. If you could, close your eyes and think of the worst nightmare that you could possibly have, one that has a horrible monster in it and the monster is chasing you. You are holding a person, one that you love so tightly, and then the monster just rips the person you love most in the world out of your arms.

". . . I live this nightmare every day. This is how I feel every day. There is no waking up and telling that person that you love them or just hold them. How could this happen to me? I do not want it to happen to you.

"Can you, just for a second, feel my fear, pain, and apprehension to go to sleep and then wake up and live it all over again, every day? It is just being so scared you want it to end. I live this nightmare every day...

"Now, we all lost his smile, his laugh, his way of having everyone in the room totally entertained and loving him for his gift of life. He brought so much laughter and love to others, why did the monster take him? Why didn't I save my son or fight for my son's life. I live this nightmare every day." (Regehr, Hill, & Glancy, 2000)

****

The authors of the following study sought to explore the degree to which Post-Traumatic Stress Symptoms (PTSS) were related to a history of SI (Suicide Ideation) and prior attempts in a national sample of firefighters ($N = 893$). They found that: "Results revealed that greater PTSS were associated with greater risk of reporting lifetime SI and prior attempts, after controlling for other known risk factors for suicidality. Exploratory models investigating the unique contributions of individual PTSS clusters to suicidality found that numbing and re-experiencing PTSS were significantly related to SI, but only re-experiencing was related to prior attempts." (Boffa et al., 2016)

****

". . . Scott had one of the most loving and caring souls that I have ever been blessed to know. Day in and day out, he would constantly ask questions as to my wellbeing and profess his love of me more times in one day than I could ever count. Whether face-to-face during normal conversations or walking up behind me, squeezeing my right shoulder, and saying, 'Love you dad;' it is something I will miss immensely.

"Suicide leaves many questions for the families, friends, and fellow firefighters. Besides wondering 'why,' survivors are sometimes left with the guilt of questioning what they missed that could have helped their loved one. They suffer from constant thoughts of why their loved one didn't ask for help.

". . . Firefighters respond to those in crisis on a daily basis and need to know that it is okay to get help as well. If firefighters feel they can't ask for help, the situation may continue to deteriorate until the result becomes tragic". (Regehr et al., 2000)

****

Summary

Essential material has emerged from recent research regarding stress loads that weaken resiliency in the aging firefighter. Among these factors are cumulative exposure to traumatic incidents, decrease in their normative sleep patterns and exposure to secondary trauma through critical incident debriefings. Considering these three contributors, I advise that critical incident debriefings be halted immediately due to the lack of scientific support for this intervention.

A definition of a critical incident was provided, followed by discussion pertaining to Critical Incident Stress Debriefing (CISD). A conclusive position on this controversial intervention was provided by the U.S. Department of Veterans Affairs – National Center for PTSD with this authoritative source noting that: "Available evidence shows that, in some instances, it may increase traumatic stress or complicate recovery."

The culture of male-dominated professions was discussed with reference to the presence of two predominant emotions. The first such sentiment is that of joviality. Words similar to this one includes festivity, gaiety, gleefulness and merriment. Often, the use or abuse of alcohol fits in perfectly with this mirthful environment.

The second primary emotion found in the male-dominated environment is that of companionate love. This is akin to 'esprit de corps' which is a feeling of pride, fellowship, and common loyalty shared by the members of a particular group.

The above emotions are positive aspects of a work environment. However, when also present in a culture of emotion suppression, work-family conflict, risk taking and health problems, stigmas emerge. When a culture of strength and power is predominant, weakness, particularly of the mental variety is strongly shunned. In a similar manner, physical weakness or illness tends to be poorly tolerated.

Unfortunately, as our firefighters age, the buildup of stress and burnout accrues. Thus, as personnel experience frustration or cynicism, there is no viable outlet available to express this in a healthy manner. As discussed, counseling is not a route that a 'macho male' would be inclined to take.

Unfortunately, even if one did voluntarily choose this path, the likely outcome would be no different given recent outcome research pertaining to 'gold standard' treatments currently utilized among the military. Hoge et. al. suggests that:

"Dropping out of care is clearly the most important predictor of treatment failure; therefore the most promising strategies to improve efficacy of evidence-based treatments will be those that address engagement, therapeutic rapport, and retention." (Hoge et al., 2014)

Thus, with few helpful outlets available, cumulative stress finds an alternative outlet and expression through psychophysiological manifestations. These were discussed in detail in the chapter and I will not elucidate further at this point. I will however, reiterate the loss of hope associated with PTSD leading to the ending of life through suicide.

I believe that there is a better way to preserve the integrity and self-esteem of those who sacrifice to keep us safe. As described in the policing chapter, change is imminent in the organization, structure and support of personnel who have dedicated their lives to protect their respective communities.

Reference List:

A Day In The Life Of Chicago's Busiest Firefighters. http://articles.chicagotribune.com/1989-03-05/news/8903240294_1_mattress-fire-truck-chicago-fire-department

Barger, L. K., Rajaratnam, S. M. W., Wang, W., O'Brien, C. S., Sullivan, J. P., Qadri, S., ... Czeisler, C. A. (2015). Common Sleep Disorders Increase Risk of Motor Vehicle Crashes and Adverse Health Outcomes in Firefighters. *Journal of Clinical Sleep*

Medicine : JCSM : Official Publication of the American Academy of Sleep Medicine, *11*(3), 233–240. https://doi.org/10.5664/jcsm.4534

Boffa, J. W., Stanley, I. H., Hom, M. A., Norr, A. M., Joiner, T. E., & Schmidt, N. B. (2016). PTSD Symptoms and Suicidal Thoughts and Behaviors among Firefighters. *Journal of Psychiatric Research*, *0*(0). https://doi.org/10.1016/j.jpsychires.2016.10.014

Critical Incident Stress. http://www.officer.com/article/10249385/critical-incident-stress

Debunking debriefing. http://articles.chicagotribune.com/2008-08-05/news/0808050478_1_school-shootings-feelings-world-trade-center

Dobson, M., Choi, B., Schnall, P. L., Wigger, E., Garcia-Rivas, J., Israel, L., & Baker, D. B. (2013). Exploring Occupational and Health Behavioral Causes of Firefighter Obesity: A Qualitative Study: Causes of Firefighter Obesity. *American Journal of Industrial Medicine*, *56*(7), 776–790. https://doi.org/10.1002/ajim.22151

Editors. (2016). Burnout: Workaholic. *Psychology Today*. Informational. https://www.psychologytoday.com/basics/burnout

Firefighter divorce: 3 important facts. http:// www .firerescue1.com/fire-rehab/articles /2181 154-Firefighter-divorce-3-important-facts/

Firefighter suicide report.pdf. http://firefighter veteran.com/images/stories/Nationla_ Volunteer_FireCounsel/Firefighter%20suici de%20report.pdf

Firefighting in Colonial America. http://www. firehouse.com/news/10527819/firefighting-in-colonial-america

Fireman Back Pain. http://www.cure-back-pain.org/fireman-back-pain.html

Harvey, S. B., Milligan-Saville, J. S., Paterson, H. M., Harkness, E. L., Marsh, A. M., Dobson, M., ... Bryant, R. A. (2016). The mental health of fire-fighters: An examination of the impact of repeated trauma exposure. *The Australian and New Zealand Journal of Psychiatry, 50*(7), 649–658. https://doi.org /10.1177/0004867415615217

Hoge, C. W., Grossman, S. H., Auchterlonie, J. L., Riviere, L. A., Milliken, C. S., & Wilk, J. E. (2014). PTSD Treatment for Soldiers After Combat Deployment: Low Utilization of Mental Health Care and Reasons for Dropout. *Psychiatric Services, 65*(8), 997–1004. https://doi.org/10.1176/appi.ps.201 300307

JMGC-Vol-3-Is-3.pdf. http://acegonline.org/wp-content/uploads/2013/02/JMGC-Vol-3-Is-3.pdf#page=5

Jones, R. L. (2001, August 29). Heart Attack Kills New Firefighter During a Blaze on Staten Island. *The New York Times*. http://www.nytimes.com/2001/08/29/nyregion/heart-attack-kills-new-firefighter-during-a-blaze-on-staten-island.html

Kales, S. N., Soteriades, E. S., Christophi, C. A., & Christiani, D. C. (2007). Emergency Duties and Deaths from Heart Disease among Fire fighters in the United States. *New England Journal of Medicine*, *356*(12), 1207–1215. https://doi.org/10.1056/NEJMoa060357

Login. http://www.fireengineering.com/login.html

Lusa, S., Miranda, H., Luukkonen, R., Punakallio, A. (2014). Sleep disturbances predict long-term changes in low back pain among Finnish firefighters: 13-year follow-up study. *International Archives of Occupa tional and Environmental Health*, *88*(3), 369–379. https://doi.org/ 10.1007/s00420-014-0968-z

NFPA report - U.S. fire department profile. http://www.nfpa.org/news-and-research/fire-statistics-and-reports/fire-statistics/the-fire-service/administration/us-fire-department-profile

O'Neill, O., & Rothbard, N. (2015). Is Love All You Need? The Effects of Emotional Culture, Suppression, and Work-family Conflict on Firefighter Risk Taking and Health. *Academy of Management Journal*, amj.2014.0952. https://doi.org/10.5465/amj.2014.0952

Pelham, B. (2016). Saving Our Heroes: A Longitudinal Study of Mental Disorders Within the Fire Service. *Scripps Senior Theses*. http://scholarship.claremont.edu/scripps_theses/774

Piazza-Gardner, A. K., Barry, A. E., Chaney, E., Dodd, V., Weiler, R., & Delisle, A. (2014). Covariates of alcohol consumption among career firefighters. *Occupational Medicine (Oxford, England)*, *64*(8), 580–582. https://doi.org/10.1093/occmed/kqu124

Post-traumatic stress disorder: The flames inside firefighters' minds. http://www.calgaryjournal.ca/index.php/news/840-post-traumatic-stress-disorder-the-flames-inside-firefighters-minds

Regehr, C., Hill, J., & Glancy, G. D. (2000). Individual predictors of traumatic reactions in firefighters. *The Journal of Nervous and Mental Disease*, *188*(6), 333–339.

Sen, S., Palmieri, T., & Greenhalgh, D. (2016). Cardiac Fatalities in Firefighters: An

Analysis of the U.S. Fire Administration Database. *Journal of Burn Care & Research: Official Publication of the American Burn Association, 37*(3), 191–195. https://doi.org/ 10.1097/BCR.000000 0000000225

Types of Debriefing Following Disasters - PTSD: National Center for PTSD. http://www.ptsd.va.gov/professional/trauma/disaster-terrorism/debriefing-after-disasters.asp

Vaulerin, J., d'Arripe-Longueville, F., Emile, M., & Colson, S. S. (2016). Physical exercise and burnout facets predict injuries in a population-based sample of French career firefighters. *Applied Ergonomics, 54*, 131–135. https://doi.org/10.1016/j.apergo.2015.12.007

Chapter Four

Emergency Medical Services

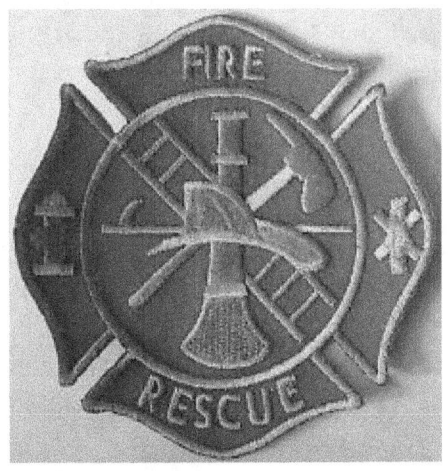

Success comes in a lot of ways, but it doesn't come with money and it doesn't come with fame. It comes from having a meaning in your life, doing what you love and being passionate about what you do. That's having a life of success. When you have the ability to do what you love, love what you do and have the ability to impact people. That's having a life of success. That's what having a life of meaning is.

Tim Tebow

The advent of the Emergency Medical System is reported to have begun during Napoleon's time to aid injured soldiers (Shah, 2006). In the US, the Civil War is credited with the emergence of a system to deal with the wounded on the field. However, the 1970's and 1980's appeared to be the primary period for the development of our current EMS that continues in use today.

The following history is longer than that provided in earlier chapters due to the relatively recent material that emerged during development of this essential component. The author of the following article perceives that through the early 1960's, the Federal Government viewed EMS primarily as a transportation agency that provided basic first aid.

"During the Civil War, the Union Army developed an organized system to evacuate soldiers from the field (Physicians, 2002)... By 1960, a patchwork of unregulated systems had developed, with services sometimes being provided by hospitals, fire departments, volunteer groups, or undertakers. Physicians staffed some ambulances, while others had minimally trained or untrained personnel. Despite the major expansion in health care facilities and the emphasis on medical specialization after World War II, the EMS system had not received much attention or innovation." (Starr, 1984).

". . . In 1960, President Kennedy announced that traffic accidents in the United States were a major public health problem needing attention (Shah, 2006). By 1965, Congressional leaders noted the large and rapidly increasing health and financial cost of trauma. This 'crisis' was occurring despite advances in trauma care that had reduced the mortality rate for injured soldiers reaching medical facilities from 4.5% during World War II to less than 2% during Vietnam.

". . . During 1965 and 1966, a convergence of political and medical actions focused the national interest on motor vehicle crashes. In 1965, President Johnson, continuing Kennedy's interest in motor vehicle crashes, created the President's Commission on Highway Safety. The Commission's report identified the great public health burden of motor vehicle crashes and stated that a coordinated national highway safety program should be a major priority.

". . . President Johnson announced his intention to discuss highway safety in his State of the Union address and transportation message in 1966. . . Simultaneously, a report released in 1966 by the National Academy of Sciences–National Research Council was extremely critical of the emergency care system. This comprehensive report, titled

'Accidental Death and Disability: The Neglected Disease of Modern Society,' documented the absence of quality emergency care.

"Some EMS-related inadequacies included: (1) no treatment protocols; (2) few trained medical personnel; (3) inefficient transportation; (4) lack of modern communications and equipment; (5) the abdication of responsibility by political authorities; and (6) the lack of research evaluating prehospital care. The recommendations of both reports were incorporated into the Highway Safety Act of 1966.

". . . The television show 'Emergency' (1971) showed EMS personnel from the Los Angeles County Fire Department heroically responding to patients suffering from traumatic and medical injuries. The EMS staff used newly developed concepts and devices such as cardiopulmonary resuscitation, defibrillation, and intravenous medications.

". . . In January 1973, Senators Cranston, Kennedy, and others reintroduced EMS legislation. Supporting arguments for the EMS Systems Development Act were made as they had been in the past. Political leaders described the crisis in public health. Senator Kennedy stated: "Nowhere is the health care crisis . . . more evident . . . than in the appalling lack of high quality emergency medical services." (Shah, 2006)

To add further complexity to the mix, EMS expressed concern related to a growing dependency on the 9-1-1 system for non-emergency medical needs. The authors of the following 2016 study reported that: ". . . the challenges of our country's poor and elderly citizens are not met by other existing safety nets. The importance of strengthening the lives and livelihoods of our vulnerable populations—and increasing their access to needed opportunities and resources—is indeed an undercurrent in this report. Currently, and often as a stopgap measure, our citizens call 9-1-1 when in need. We would be wise to heed the concerns of the men and women who respond to those calls." (Cannuscio et al., 2016)

The structure/framework for this chapter will consist of the following components: job description; job tempo, family; special incidents; employee burnout; stress effects and their association with PTSD; suicide.

****

"15.109 . . . I don't know what triggered it, but I woke up one day and decided that I didn't want to go to work anymore, so I called in sick . . . but in reality I sat at home drinking all day and then struggling to find sleep at night, tossing and turning until I drank enough to make me pass out. I suddenly dreaded the thought of having to go back, and I dropped into an absolutely black pit of depression. . .

"I found myself sitting in a lobby filling out a form with check boxes for symptoms I was experiencing while I waited to be seen . . .

"She told me that I qualified as likely suffering from PTSD and handed me a brochure about dealing with it. She said, apologetically, that due to a large volume of patients, the only available options for me during the next year were group counseling for PTSD and another referral, this time for a psychiatrist who could give me an anti-depressant. She added, if I liked, I could reserve a place in line to receive individual counseling, but the waiting list was 10 to 12 months.

"To say that I was taken aback doesn't fully encompass the anger I felt, followed by the crushing feeling that I would have to wait a year before I could talk to someone. . .

"My meeting with the HMO psychiatrist was even worse than having the initial evaluation done, if that's possible. It lasted about 5 minutes, during which the doc looked over my form from the psych eval, tallied up the score again and said he could offer me 10 ativan and an antidepressant, just as advertised.

"That was it. No questions, no 'how are you doing', he just looked at my score and sent me off with a tiny dose of Celexa that wouldn't calm a squirrel and a couple of ativan. He offered no follow up plan, no other referrals, and not even a handshake. So I left." ("About," 2015)

****

Emergency medical services (EMS), includes a range of personnel who have obtained differing levels of certification. For example, the most common type of providers in this group are Emergency Medical Technicians (EMTs) who are the entry-level patient care provider. These are followed by EMT-Intermediates and then paramedics. The following descriptions are from a UCLA article that describes the differences between the EMT and Paramedic.

The author reports that: "EMTs learn the essential skills to help in life-threatening situations and their education is the foundation for all other levels of provider. . . Both EMTs and paramedics have the knowledge and skills to transport patients and provide them with emergency care. The biggest difference between them is the amount of education they receive and what they are allowed to do for patients (scope of practice).

"EMT's usually complete a course that is about 120-150 hours in length. In contrast, paramedic courses can be between 1,200 to 1,800 hours. EMT and paramedic courses consist of lectures, hands-on skills training, and clinical and/or field internships.

"EMTs are educated in many skills including CPR, giving patients oxygen, administering glucose for diabetics, and helping others with treatments for asthma attacks or allergic reactions. With very few exceptions, such as in the case of auto-injectors for allergic reactions, EMTs are not allowed to provide treatments that requiring breaking the skin: that means no needles.

"Paramedics are advanced providers of emergency medical care and are highly educated in topics such as anatomy and physiology, cardiology, medications, and medical procedures. They build on their EMT education and learn more skills such as administering medications, starting intravenous lines, providing advanced airway management for patients, and learning to resuscitate and support patients with significant problems such as heart attacks and traumas. Paramedic education programs may last six to twelve months ("What's the Difference Between an EMT and a Paramedic?" | UCLA CPC," n.d.)

The tempo/pace of the job is similar to that of the fireman in that there are periods of routine followed by inactivity interrupted by bursts of demand. This is punctuated by occasional critical incidents mixed with uneventful calls. The following example typifies a day in an EMT's on call experiences:

****

"EMT Wendy Cureall starts her 24-hour shift at midnight. . . The call is for a collapsed elderly male at a private residence. . . A police officer at the door directs her upstairs. . . He is conscious and turns his head to face Wendy, which causes her stress level to fall dramatically. Luke and one of the police officers carefully move Hector to the ground floor using a stair chair. There, they transfer him to the stretcher that Wendy has brought from the rig.

". . . the radio alarm goes off. The 911 dispatcher . . . requesting a transport for a patient with dehydration. . . The smell as they enter is overwhelming. It is obvious why the patient . . . is dehydrated. She has been suffering from diarrhea in her bed for who knows how long.

"When they arrive back at the station, the dispatcher calls them out to an MVA (motor vehicle accident) . . . Upon arriving at the scene, they find a young female driver behind the wheel of a subcompact. Apparently, she didn't see the back of the tractor trailer truck stopped in front of her. (Want to bet she was texting?) . . .The firefighters arrive to remove the car door and they help the EMTs to put the driver onto a spineboard and move her into the rig. . . The rest of the shift is uneventful." ("EMT: Typical Day," n.d.)

****

The National Association of State EMS Officials (NASEMSO) revealed that: ". . . there are 78,258 credentialed EMS vehicles in the U.S., or three for every 10,000 people. . . 30 professional EMS responders (are available) per 10,000 of people. . . For 2009, there were an estimated 36,698,670 EMS events (responses) in the U.S., resulting in approximately 28,004,624 transports." (By, 2011)

In regard to wages, the US Bureau of Labor Statistics report that: "The median annual wage for EMTs and paramedics was $31,980 in May 2015... The lowest 10 percent earned less than $20,860, and the highest 10 percent earned more than $55,110... Most paid EMTs and paramedics work full time. About 1 in 3 worked more than 40 hours per week in 2014. Because EMTs and paramedics must be available to work in emergencies, they may work overnight and on weekends. Some EMTs and paramedics work shifts in 12- or 24-hour increments." ("EMTs and Paramedics," n.d.)

The system is decentralized, with training, protocols, organizational climate, and social context varying . . . the fire service has become an important out-of-hospital source of emergency medical care. Indeed, nearly half of the nation's EMS systems are based in fire departments." (Cannuscio et al., 2016)

I find that the absence of wellness and prevention programs for EMS professionals as discussed in the NASEMSO article to be a point of concern particularly within the context of the following material: "The United States is experiencing a severe shortage of Emergency Medical Service (EMS) paramedics. The job outlook for paramedics (EMT-P) for the years 2012-2022 is predicted to increase by 23%-33%, which is much faster than the 4% average increase of other first-response professions. The average tenure of paramedics is less than 4 years." (Paschal, 2016)

The four-year average tenure has apparently led some researchers to look for the 'ideal' personality type that is the best fit for the job. Apparently, when identified, this type will be able to unaffectedly provide a career of service maintaining efficiency throughout their tenure.

As discussed in earlier chapters, the issue of the 'ideal personality' for the profession continues to be investigated. I would propose that the direction of this research misses the critical point pertaining to the increasing toll that cumulative stress and trauma has on EMS staff. The position I have taken, as stated in earlier chapters, is that independent of personality style or attachment aspects, cumulative exposure to critical incidents leads to burnout in our EMS personnel.

****

"15.96 ". . . I have became distant from a lot of people, easily agitated and upset. some of this resulted in things like me forgetting stuff or starting on something and just going off and not finishing it. It seems like all I want to do anymore is just be alone and lay on the couch.

"All of this has affected my personal life. I used to love going out and having fun. . . I kept everything to myself instead of talking about things and decompressing. I was slowly turning into someone I didn't know.

"I did go to therapy, it did not seem to help, yes I talked openly to my therapist, but in the end all they did was prescribe me medications that made me feel like a zombie, and then it turned to changing medications every month to the point i was feeling physically sick, i was going days without eating or sleeping, the anxiety and depression only got worse.

"I went through 3 different therapists in under a year, and all 3 seemed more focused on medications that in the end made me feel worse. All this made for a decline in my relationship with my girlfriend, i kept quiet about how i felt, i was always more concerned about her then i was myself i didn't want her to have to worry about me all the time.

"... All these things i never realized until a friend/coworker committed suicide recently. It was and still is very hard for me to deal with because it reminded me a lot of the situations i was in the past few years and how close i was to having the same ending." ("About," 2015)

****

Recent research suggests that the families of EMS personnel are not free from the effects of secondary PTSD among their loved one. The author of the following study has found that: "... The images and feelings that are associated with continuously being exposed to traumatic situations are not limited to the emergency services personnel, who are primarily exposed to the event, but these events can also have an effect on the significant others in their environment, such as their spouses. The aim of this study was to explore and describe the experiences of secondary trauma among the spouses of emergency services personnel.

"... The data was collected by means of semi-structured individual interviews ... The experiences of secondary trauma among the spouses of emergency services personnel stemmed from their partners' repeated exposure to trauma, managing everyday job stress, safety fears, behavioural changes, dealing with their partners' emotional reactivity and emotional withdrawal from the family, following trauma exposure." (Wheater, 2016)

****

"15.84: When you think about suicide in fire /ems you have to wonder what would cause someone take such a permanent step. I think what happened to me will shed some light on this problem. I have been a paramedic on our fire department for 21 and 1/2 years. I never had any problems for most of my time there. All of that changed the day a 13 year old girl died in an MVA, and we were unable to get her out.

"A switch was flipped and everything changed from than on. I am unable to sleep at night anymore as I get 'visited' by this girl and many others that have died since. It grew worse and I began to feel there was no way to stop it. . . I started to see people every-where look like they had blood all over their head and face. I was losing it fast.

"One day I found myself in a place where I could not deal with it anymore. I saw no way out. I went to work that morning and was going to hang myself in my room at the fire hall. I was going to do this at work because I did not want my family to find me. I was broken.

"We got a run and I had to take it before I could even get to my room. It's amazing to think I am still alive because of that run. They pulled me off the truck that morning and asked me if I needed help. I now had to make a choice. Go back to the hall and end the nightmare, or seek help and start to fight. I chose to get help. That began a three month fight to try and keep my career.

"Because PTSD is not recognized I found myself losing all of my saved up vacation days. I fought every office the department could throw at me to try and keep my days. In the end it was a losing battle and I ran out of time. I am getting help.

"The MD and therapist I am seeing refuse to clear me to go back because I tried to take my own life. Now I have run out of time and I find myself on the outside looking in. My 22 year career is gone." ("About," 2015)

****

Special circumstances are to be occasionally expected within the first responder's routine. One such situation is that of dealing with the mentally ill when responding to a call. The authors of the following 2015 study suggest that: ". . . Despite the frequent involvement of EMS with people with mental health and substance abuse problems, the nature and content of this work, as well as how EMS providers think about this work, have not been fully explored.

"Using data obtained through observations and interviews with providers at an urban American EMS agency, this paper provides an analysis of the ways in which EMS providers interact with people with mental illness and substance abuse problems, as well as providers' experiences with the mental health care system.

"Results demonstrate that EMS providers share common beliefs and frustrations about 'psych calls' and the types of calls that involve people with behavioral health problems. In addition, providers described their understandings of the ways in which people with mental health and substance use problems 'abuse the system' and the consequences of this abuse." (Prener & Lincoln, 2015)

Another circumstance of concern is that of violence directed towards EMS and other first responder personnel. The author of the following article noted that: "Over two-thirds of EMS personnel experienced at least one form of violence in the last 12 months." (Gormley, Crowe, Bentley, & Levine, 2016)

An earlier study (2012) referred to how 'victim incivility' might have on the emergency service employee. The author found that: ". . . The results showed that victim incivility predicted exhaustion, physical symptoms, and absenteeism. Additionally, both engagement and empathy buffered some negative outcomes, although empathy actually exacerbated the negative effects of victim incivility on absenteeism." (Sliter, 2012)

Finally, incidents involving injured children appears to universally affect rescue personnel worldwide because so many have an emotional connection with the victim. The authors of the following 2015 article note that: ". . . Although EMS personnel are trained and prepared to deal with the technical aspects of incidents they will face in their career, they are less prepared to manage the psychological impact of these events.

"Participants used avoidance as a coping mechanism by focusing on patient management and the anatomy, physiology and pathology related to the patient's condition within their relevant scope of practice and treatment. By doing this, they reduce the risk of developing an emotional connection with the patient.

"Talking to their colleagues after the incident was a key coping mechanism and acted as an informal debriefing tool. This method of debriefing and getting confirmation that their patient care was correct contributes a great deal to their ability to cope with the trauma.

"Most participants indicated that they had received little or no training to prepare them for the emotional effects of traumatic incidents or how to deal with the bereaved family. . . The attitude of 'boys don't cry' in EMS might hinder personnel to contact . . . other available support structures.

"They do not show their emotions because they have to maintain the image of being the provider, protect their reputation of being strong, and do not want people to think that they are weak when they show that an incident has affected them emotionally." (Minnie, Goodman, & Wallis, 2015)

In regard to EMS burnout, a 2016 study provided a comprehensive overview of personal, work related and patient related burnout. The author notes that: "About one-third (33.8%) of EMTs and paramedics were classified as having personal burnout. Over one-quarter (26.3%) met the criteria for work-related burnout and 11.1% had patient-related burnout. Slightly less than a quarter (21.1%) of EMTs and paramedics said that they would likely leave their current main EMS jobs within the next 12 months. . . Finally, a total of 3.4% of EMTs and paramedics reported missing 10 or more days of work due to sickness in the past 12 months.

". . . After controlling for other covariates, paramedics had greater odds of both personal and patient-related burnout than EMTs. . . With regards to years of EMS experience, compared to those with fewer than 5 years of experience, those in the middle range of between 5 and 15 years of EMS experience had greater odds of work-related burnout.

". . . Those at private agencies had greater odds of work-related burnout compared to those at fire-based agencies. These results are supported by a study that found that those working at private agencies had a 35% increase in odds of stress compared to those at fire-based agencies.

". . . Weekly call volume was the only significant predictor of all three dimensions of burnout. The odds of burnout in each dimension were greatest for those who reported having more than 20 calls per week." ("!etd.pdf," 2017)

An emerging pattern that holds true for EMT, as well as police and firefighter personnel, is that cumulative trauma experiences produce burnout, ultimately leading to PTSD symptoms in many of those who serve and protect. A 2016 study focused on the high-stress environment and exposure to critical incidents among EMS personnel.

The investigators provided: "An online survey administered to . . . EMS providers. Of the 2,683 respondents, more than one quarter (27.7%) met the PTSD criteria of 50 or higher on the PCL-M. Close to half of the respondents (42.0%) reported having contemplated suicide in the last six months.

". . . nearly one third (27.1%) thought about suicide 10 or more days in the last 30 days. . . PTSD scores and suicide ideation frequency were highest when post-incident services were not available in the workplace." (Boldt, 2016)

When EMT staff reach a level of dysfunction as descried in the earlier study, there is little question that it is going to affect their job performance. This is evident in the following 2016 study: "A sample of 134 (103 male, 31 female) rural and regional ambulance personnel completed a mixed methods survey assessing fatigue, stress and emotional trauma. . . Participants reported high levels of fatigue and emotional trauma.

"Qualitative data revealed stressors including community expectations and 'office politics'. Participants also reported negative effects of fatigue including errors in drug administration and falling asleep while driving." (Pyper & Paterson, 2016)

Media coverage of a number of fire departments including Phoenix, Arizona, Chicago, Illinois and Montgomery County, Maryland investigated suicide incidents among their staff. "The Phoenix (AZ) Fire department lost four firefighters who committed suicide in a seven-month period.

"The Chicago (IL) Fire department lost 37 firefighters to suicide since tracking this method of death, and the Montgomery County (MD) Fire department reported the loss of 17 firefighters to suicide in the past 13 years.

"Recent statistics collected by Jeff Dill, director and licensed counselor of the counseling Services for Fire Fighters, reports that more than 160 firefighters committed suicide since 2000. Preliminary analysis shows firearms was the most used method, followed by hanging, carbon monoxide poisoning, and overdose. ongoing data collection may reveal the numbers are even higher once reporting and tracking mechanisms become formalized.

"We could continue to list the other individual suicides impacting career, call, and volunteer fire departments across the country. The fire service, like many other areas of the workforce, is faced with members returning from serving on the front line of a war.

"How the fire service integrates returning veterans to the department can play a significant role in the veterans' mental health. it is important to note that a majority of military firefighters deployed to Iraq and Afghanistan are reservists and guardsmen and paid and volunteer firefighters when in civilian status, and they return to civilian departments after multiple deployments." ("FEU-AntonellisDec12.pdf," 2012)

We can and must end the hopelessness and despair occurring to our vital frontline service personnel who are there for us in our time of need. There is a way to prevent the buildup of cumulative stress effects. Now is the time to implement this life saving intervention.

Summary

Abuse of the 9-1-1 system has become an issue of concern among EMS staff. The tempo of EMS is similar to that of the firefighting service in regard to the nature of calls, rituals and times of inactivity. The estimate of increasing need for paramedics ranging from 23%-33% mixed with the average tenure of less than 4 years (Paschal, 2016) is clearly an area of concern. An intervention to block the buildup of cumulative stress in this occupational group clearly is in the best interest of the communities they serve.

Research into the 'ideal' personality type is ongoing although in my opinion is rather fruitless. I don't believe there is a personality type, other that perhaps the sociopathic, that can be unaffected over the long run by the tragedies encountered within the context of daily service.

Indeed, the secondary trauma effects on the family of EMS personnel has become a topic of recent research. A 2013 article supported the hypothesis that stress and burnout experienced by paramedics in the work setting predicted subsequent outcomes in the home setting for both paramedics and their spouses.

Special circumstances were discussed including: the handling of patients with mental illnesses; verbal or physical violence expressed towards EMS personnel with over 2/3 experiencing this phenomenon within a 12-month period. The handling of incidents involving children are universally difficult for EMS staff to handle.

The primary way that the service member deals with issues of concern is to discuss matters with their colleagues, as opposed to seeking professional intervention. As exemplified in the included 'stories', when profession intervention is sought it frequently ends up with a dissatisfied client/patient. Varied studies reveal high levels of burnout among EMS staff culminating in typical longevity of around 4 years of service. This pattern appears to be strongly associated with the number of calls handled on a weekly basis.

Negative impact on job performance has been reported when calls per week meet or exceed 20 per week. When this occurs, errors in drug administration and falling asleep while driving have been reported." (Pyper & Paterson, 2016) Finally, the incidence of suicide among firefighters, which include EMS staff, tends to be under reported due to a number of factors. Among these variables is the reality that many returning military with unresolved

PTSD proceed to enter into first responder positions. Then, the cumulative effects of trauma add to the alteration in personality that is too frequently evidenced among EMS personnel.

Reference List:

About. http://codegreencampaign.org/

Boldt, F. (2016). The Relationship between Personal Factors, Work Factors, PTSD, and Suicide Ideation in Emergency Medical Service Providers. *Masters Theses & Specialist Projects.* http://digitalcommons. wku.edu /theses/1625

By, B. T. Y. NASEMSO Survey Provides Snapshot of EMS Industry. http://www .jems.com /articles /2011/11/nasemso-survey-provides-snapshot-ems-ind.html

Cannuscio, C. C., Davis, A. L., Kermis, A. D., Khan, Y., Dupuis, R., & Taylor, J. A. (2016). A Strained 9-1-1 System and Threats to Public Health. *Journal of Community Health, 41,* 658–666. https://doi.org/10.1007/s10900-015-0142-x

EMT: Typical Day. http://www.shmoop.com/ careers /emt/typical-day.html

EMTs and Paramedics : Occupational Outlook Handbook: : U.S. Bureau of Labor Statistics. http://www.bls.gov/ooh/healthcare/emts-and-paramedics.htm#tab-5

!etd.pdf. https://etd.ohiolink.edu/!etd.send _file?acces sion=osu145224540& disposition=attachment

FEU-AntonellisDec12.pdf. http://www.fireengine ering.com/content/dam/fe/online-articles/ documents/FEU/FEU-AntonellisDec12.pdf

Gormley, M. A., Crowe, R. P., Bentley, M. A., & Levine, R. (2016). A National Description of Violence toward Emergency Medical Ser-vices Personnel. *Prehospital Emergency Care: Official Journal of the National Association of EMS Physicians and the National Association of State EMS Directors*, *20*(4), 439–447. https:/ /doi.org/10.3109 /10903127.2015.1128029

Minnie, L., Goodman, S., & Wallis, L. (2015). Exposure to daily trauma: The experiences and coping mechanism of Emergency Medical Personnel. A cross-sectional study. *African Journal of Emergency Medicine*, *5*(1), 12–18. https:// doi.org/10.1016/ j.afjem.2014 .10.010

Paschal, B. (2016). 16PF® Traits as Predictors of Emer gency Medical Service Worker Tenure. *Walden Dissertations and Doctoral Studies*. http:// scholarworks.waldenu.edu/dissertations/2226

Physicians, N. A. of E. (2002). *Prehospital Systems and Medical Oversight: National Association of EMS Physicians* (3rd edition). Dubuque, Iowa: Kendall Hunt Publishing Co.

Prener, C., & Lincoln, A. K. (2015). Emergency medical services and "psych calls": Examining the work of urban EMS providers. *The American Journal of Orthopsychiatry*, *85*(6), 612–619. https://doi .org/10.1037 /ort0000077

Pyper, Z., & Paterson, J. L. (2016). Fatigue and mental health in Australian rural and regional ambulance personnel. *Emergency Medicine Australasia: EMA*, *28*(1), 62–66. https://doi.org/10.1111/1742-6723.12520

Shah, M. N. (2006). The Formation of the Emer-gency Medical Services System. *American Journal of Public Health*, *96*(3), 414–423. https://doi.org/10.2105/ AJPH.2004.048793

Sliter, M. T. (2012). *But We're Here to Help! Positive Buffers of the Relationship between Victim Incivility and Employee Outcomes in Firefighters*. Bowling Green State University. https://etd.ohiolink.edu/pg_10?0::NO:10:P10_ACCESSION_NUM:bgsu1338682142

Starr, P. (1984). *The Social Transformation of American Medicine: The rise of a sovereign profession and the making of a vast industry* (Reprint edition). New York: Basic Books.

What's the Difference Between an EMT and a Paramedic? | UCLA CPC. https://www.cpc.mednet.ucla.edu/node/27

Wheater, K. L. (2016). Spouses' experience of secondary trauma among emergency services personnel. http://etd.uwc.ac.za/xmlui/handle/11394/5004

Chapter Five

Nursing

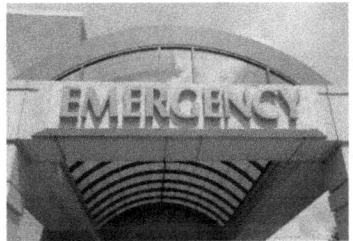

"I have an almost complete disregard of precedent, and a faith in the possibility of something better. It irritates me to be told how things have always been done. I defy the tyranny of precedent. I go for anything new that might improve the past."

Clara Barton

"As caretakers of children, family and community, it was natural that women were the nurses, the caregivers, as human society evolved. Nursing may be the oldest known profession, as some nurses were paid for their services from the beginning. . . Even when the nation's first hospital began in Philadelphia in 1751, it was thought of primarily as an asylum or poorhouse; another century or more would pass before the public viewed hospitals as reputable and safe.

"The Civil War gave enormous impetus to the building of hospitals and to the development of nursing as a credentialed profession. . . Some women had the courage and common sense to defy decorum, . . . The best known of these women, of course, is Clara Barton (who) . . . herself acknowledged that she actually nursed for only about six months of the four-year war and that other women did much more.

"Perhaps the best-known nurse at the time, was Mary Ann Bickerdyke of Illinois. . . After witnessing suffering soldiers who had literally no one to care for them, she went on to be the only woman that General William T. Sherman allowed with his army.

"In the Confederacy, the most prominent nurses were Captain Sally Tompkins and Phoebe Pember. Tompkins . . . converted her Richmond mansion into Robertson Hospital and established a reputation for extraordinary quality: Tompkins' hospital had by far the lowest death rate of any facility in the North or South, even though physicians sent their worst cases to her . . . Her staff of six . . . treated more than 1,600 patients and lost only 73, an uncommonly low number in an era before germ theory was understood.

"Phoebe Levy Pember . . . A young widow from a wealthy, Jewish family . . . went north to the Confederate capital of Richmond and eventually ran the world's largest hospital. On an average day, Pember supervised the treatment of 15,000 patients, most of them cared for by nearly 300 slave women.

". . . Often called 'sisters' (as British nurses still are), their lives were indeed similar to those of nuns. Forbidden to marry, they were cloistered in 'nurses' homes' on hospital grounds, where every aspect of life was strictly disciplined." ("Support - National Women's History Museum - NWHM," 2010)

As utilized in prior chapters, the framework for this chapter will consist of the following components:

job description; job tempo; employee burnout; family stress impact; special incidents; stress effects and their association with PTSD; medication abuse among nurses; suicide.

"Emergency Nurses treat patients in emergency situations where they're experiencing trauma or injury. These nurses quickly recognize life-threatening problems and are trained to help solve them on the spot. They can work in hospital emergency rooms, ambulances, helicopters, urgent care centers, sports arenas, and more." ("Emergency Nurse," n.d.)

Furthermore, as noted in the following article: "Registered nurses usually take one of three education paths: a bachelor's degree in nursing, an associate's degree in nursing, or a diploma from an approved nursing program. Registered nurses must also be licensed. . . Employment of registered nurses is projected to grow 19 percent from 2012 to 2022, faster than the average for all occupations.

"Growth will occur for a number of reasons, including an increased emphasis on preventative care; growing rates of chronic conditions, such as diabetes and obesity; and demand for healthcare services from the baby boomer population, as they live longer and more active lives.

". . . The average national salary of jobs for this career was $64,000 with a high confidence ranking based on over 250 sources. Average Registered Nurse salaries for job postings nationwide are 7% higher than average salaries for all job postings nationwide. . . The top 10 percent in the field earn over $94,000." (http://nursejournal.org, 2017)

Generally, these professionals have many years of experience, and usually have their master's degree in nursing. The following article describes the work conditions and environment that the newly graduating nurse is entering into.

The authors report that: "In 2009, the American College of Emergency Physicians released the National Report Card on the State of Emergency Medicine and "access to emergency care" receiving a "D". The reason for this dismal grade is the fact that the nation has too few emergency departments to meet the needs of a growing and aging population.

Over the past 10 years, the number of people needing emergency care annually has increased 32%, from 90.3 million to 119.2 million. At the same time, the number of hospital emergency departments in the country has dropped nearly 7%, from 4,109 to 3,833." ("recentworkforcestudies nov09.pdf," 2011)

Another article related to shortages in the emergency medicine workforce was published in 2009 in Annals of Emergency Medicine. In 2006, the IOM released a series of three reports on the future of emergency medicine concluding that emergency departments and ambulatory services are overburdened, under-funded, and highly fragmented.

"Patients face long waits in overcrowded emergency rooms and often needed on-call specialists are not available. A significant contributing factor is that more and more patients are turning to emergency departments for care because of lack of insurance, for after-hours care, or due to limited options in rural communities"("https://www.aamc.org/download /100 598 / data/," 2012)

****

"When I went from being a firefighter paramedic and working 24 hour shifts to being a nurse and working 12 hour shifts, probably the biggest surprise to me was the fact that working a 12 hour shift is as mentally and sometimes physically taxing as working a 24.

"That's because as a nurse, you don't get 'down time' in between patients. You always have at least one, usually more, and you are always thinking ahead to what has been done, what still needs to be done, who is sitting in triage and will probably be your next patient and what will be need to be done immediately for that patient, and so on...for 12 hours. Now, I've worked 24 hour shifts and worked two jobs at a time for nearly 20 years, but this is without a doubt the most stressful job I've ever done.

"Add to that the fact that our administration is wasting- hundreds of thousands of dollars on 'consulting groups' to *supposedly* increase our productivity, and we are in a constant state of flux because of that, and there are now constant and unrelenting pressures on us to produce as though we were assembly line workers pumping out auto parts, and you can maybe understand that my level of stress has been bumped up by more than a few notches in the last eight months or so." ("A stressed-out ER nurse tells her story." 2013)

****

Since the passage of the Affordable Care Act (ACA) in 2010, over 30 million people who were previously uninsured have the chance to be covered. What this means to ER nursing staff is that patient overcrowding and understaffing due to burned out colleagues adds to the burden.

Furthermore, it is estimated that required paperwork associated with the billing requires an estimated 190 million hours of extra paperwork every year. Within the context of a 'stressed system,' increased levels of sick days are taken, numbers of medical errors increase and the quality of patient care diminishes. (!"2013-3rded-advocacyhandbook-interactive.pdf," n.d.-b 2013)

The term boarding is referenced in the following article and therefore a definition of the label is in order. Boarding is: after admission to the hospital, because of unavailability of hospital beds or critical ER staff, the patient is held in the emergency department (often on a gurney) until help or space is available.

"Emergency department crowding, a problem that arises when the number of patients exceeds the treatment space capacity, is a national epidemic... Even though most Americans have seen and/or heard of crowding and boarding – overflowing waiting rooms, long wait times, and patients on gurneys in the hallway or tucked into corners, to name just a few examples – there is no one more attuned to the dangers and frustrations of this pervasive problem than those who work in the emergency department.

". . . While ED visits have increased, there has been a corresponding decline in the number of emergency departments. In the last 20 years, the number of emergency departments decreased from 5,108 to 4,564 . . . overall inpatient bed numbers also have decreased over the past 30 years, going from 1.36 million inpatient beds in 1981 to 941,995 in 2010.

". . . There is significant concern for actual patient harm from boarding. Patients with acute coronary syndromes who experience a delay in care may face a significant increase in death, cardiac arrest, heart failure, arrhythmia, and hypotension during times of crowding. . .

"Increases in medical errors are associated with boarding, such as missing a dose of home medication or a missed ED treatment; these are errors of omission (not commission), precipitated by the simultaneous care of inpatients and new emergency patients." (!"2013-3rded-advocacy handbook -inter-ative.pdf," n.d.-b 2013)

The preceding information certainly appears to be challenging within the context of providing quality ER services. To further complicate matters, we add the human factor to the mix by exploring the first hour in an emergency nurse's 12-hour shift. The author reports that after taking report from the off-going shift:

****

". . . We're interrupted by an Emergency Medical Services EMS crew coming in the door with an intoxicated male, wearing Siamese friendship bracelets (handcuffs), who needs jail clearance. The police tried to help him find his family to take him home, but he was so belligerent to the police that he talked his way into jail. . .

"Shaggy, bearded mid 40's male, who has wet his pants. He's a frequent flier, so I know him by name, know his medical history, and who usually comes for him if he's behaved and can go home sober. . . Mental note: bet the new doc that Shaggy's blood alcohol will be around .320—legal is less that, at .080. I get lots of free sodas that way and experienced staff won't bet me anymore.

"A registration clerk . . . asks me to check on a car outside the front door. Mama has 2 children at home and number 3 has just arrived on the car floor. The nursing assistant brings some supplies (how do they always know what's needed before I do?). I quickly wrap the baby and clamp the cord noting the time carefully for the birth certificate.

". . . On the way, I ask the police watching Shaggy if they want coffee. . . I finally have time to make a route past the coffee machine to my computer terminal, and I take a sip of coffee as I log on to catch up with my patient's orders. A quick glance at my watch tells me I've still got 11 more hours left to be an emergency room nurse." ("A Day in the Life of an Emergency Room Nurse," 2016)

****

As noted in the above article, the ER pace is rapid, often hectic at times and filled with a wide variation of often challenging circumstances. We shall explore some of these influences beginning with the following 2016 article wherein the author proposes that self-compassion may be a protective factor mitigating against the long-term effects of burnout and ultimately of PTSD in the ER environment:

"The main goal of this study was to explore how empathy and self-compassion related to professional quality of life (compassion satisfaction, compassion fatigue and burnout). . . Teaching self-compassion and self-care skills may be an important feature in interventions that aim to reduce burnout and compassion fatigue." (J. Duarte, Pinto-Gouveia, & Cruz, 2016)."

I wonder how one teaches self-caring and self-compassion within the madness of a fully engaged ER setting. Is this a quality that is able to be exercised over the entire course of a 12-hour shift in a highly volatile environment? I doubt it. Personally, I'm not the same individual I was at the end of a harrowing day than I was when the day began.

Isn't compassion a necessary quality for ER personnel? I perceive that rather than focusing on self-compassion in the midst of a whirlwind, the proper quest is one of finding a way to be able to avoid carrying the horrific experiences of today into tomorrow. The nurse in the following story clearly has been unable to accomplish this objective.

****

"I found myself saying, 'I love the ER, but I kinda hate people now.' And that makes me sad. I started this career as a nice person, one who loves people and helping them and was full of naivete and compassion... When I get a patient who says to me, 'I hurt which works for me is Dilaudid,' instead of thinking she hurts really bad and has been through this be- fore I immediately jump to how much of a drug seeker she must be and how it's bullshit to even be in the ER right now.

"When a 22 year old comes in the ambulance for a mild asthma exacerbation, texting and wearing a brand new hat, then asked for a cab voucher home, I don't think that perhaps he's homeless and wearing the only things of value he has in the world; instead I think he's just a typical arrogant entitled drain on society who will get that voucher because the hospital can't say no without getting a bad review.

"When a patient lashes out at me and calls me horrible names, instead of thinking that he is in the most stressful time of his life. . .

I immediately write him off as a horrible person and provide appropriate nursing care but extend only the bare minimum of servility to him... I never wanted to be that cynical nurse from the nursing school horror stories... I'm hoping the system will someway start to be fixed, because seriously. This can't continue." (Shrtstormtrooper, 2014)

****

An earlier study (2015) investigated the level of burnout of clinical nurses by examining varied factors contributing to this phenomenon. The researchers found that: "... The participants had moderate levels of emotional exhaustion ... and depersonalization ... and a high level of reduced personal accomplishment.

"Both personal and environmental factors were correlated with nurse burnout; however, personal factors played bigger roles in predicting personal accomplishment, whereas environmental factors played bigger roles in predicting emotional exhaustion and depersonalization." (Wang, Liu, & Wang, 2015)

Candidly, I don't fully comprehend the above reference. I'm guessing that 'personal factors' pertain to matters outside of the work setting. But then, when one comes home from an impossible shift, how could it not affect the home environment? The associated issue of moral distress often accompanies the burnout phenomena as noted in the following reference:

"Sources of moral distress identified included patient advocacy issues, professional behavior of other health care professionals, internal conflicts with what they perceived to be the right thing to do and that which was asked of them, and guilt over their own feelings about patient care." (Robinson & Stinson, 2016)

The prior material also leads to our discussion of the adverse effects of medical errors on the involved ER personnel. When the incident is severe, typically an investigation results that can have serious consequences on the ability of the 'secondary victims' (involved nursing personnel) to continue to practice. An English study estimates a "10.4 - 43.3% prevalence of second victims after an adverse event."

The authors of the study further postulate that: "The fate of practitioners who have blown the whistle in the interest of patient safety and have paid with their livelihood, health, and/or family life is very closely linked to the issues discussed in this report. . . Suicides associated with incidents and investigations do happen, but the extent of the problem essentially remains hidden, as not all organisations are able to identify them with confidence." ("FINAL REPORT Suicides by clinicians involved in SIs in the NHS.pdf," 2014)

****

"The nurse grabbed the recliner, jerking me awake. 'Leilani, you have to get up!' I heard Code Blue and the room filled with people. In that instant, I knew he was gone. The next hours were awful – my sweet, joyful boy had become a corpse hooked to machines. . . My 20-month old son had just died in one of the country's leading hospitals.

"When he was admitted to the hospital, white circles with wires were stuck to Gabriel's bare chest to monitor his breathing and heartbeat. Every time he made the slightest wiggle the alarms went off. . . We had already spent sleepless days and nights in my hometown hospital in Reno where Gabriel had been misdiagnosed again and again. . . But now we were at Stanford's hospital for children.

"Finally, I felt safe. And very tired. I am sure the nurse could see how tired I was. She wanted to take care of me too, so she . . . turned off the sound on the alarms next to Gabriel's bed. I thanked her when she did it. I was so grateful for the prospect of sleep.

"Later, doctors and administrators would tell me that she had unknowingly done a lot more.

"She . . . had turned off all the alarms everywhere . . . So when Gabriel's heart stopped beating there was no sound, just quiet. Nothing woke me until the nurse found him. . . He died at a hospital that had people brave enough to face me, bold enough to take responsibility, compassionate enough to explain. Because of this, I am one of the lucky ones." ("I Am One of the Lucky Ones: A Mother's Story of Medical Error," 2014)

****

I've included the following 2016 article as followup to the prior discussion. The author's purpose was to "explore the benefit of recognizing the signs and symptoms of burnout, introduce interventions to combat PTSD, and improve resiliency in ED RNs." Unfortunately, the perception still remains that critical incident stress debriefing (CISD) is still a viable intervention for improving resiliency even though it has been discredited in recent scientific literature.

"The use of the wounded healer theory provides a framework to help nurse managers develop strategies such as critical incident stress debriefing (CISD) to address emotional distress." ("Hidden Grief and Lasting Emotions in Emergency Department Nurses: Ingenta Connect," 2016)

A variety of special incidents are briefly reviewed in this section. I have numbered and will discuss the following matters as elucidated in a 2009 dissertation by Cynthia Francis Bechtel who categorizes critical incidents in the following manner:

"A moral distress event resulted when interference from family or coworkers prevented emergency nurses from fulfilling their duties (1), potentially leading to a critical incident for emergency nurses. When a lack of responsiveness by a healthcare professional, such as a physician (2), occurred that affected patient care, it could create a critical incident for nurses. Emergency situations that involved cardiac or respiratory arrests (3) could precipitate critical incident stress. Lastly, exposure to potentially infectious materials (4) created a critical incident stress situation for the nurses because of fear of developing disease.

"Critical incidents have been defined as events that potentially overwhelm a nurse' usual coping skills and produce unusual distress in a healthy person. Critical incidents identified most frequently by nurses include: the death of a child (5), injury, or abuse of a child (6)." ("Emergency Nursesâ•Ž Experiences with Critical Incidents: A Dissertation - viewcontent. cgi, 2016)

Also, a primary difficulty encountered in the ER environment is the issue of violence manifested against ER personnel. A study utilizing 5,000 nurses from a US urban/community hospital system was conducted which revealed the following data:

". . . investigated the incidence of workplace violence against nurses perpetrated by patients or visitors in their hospital system. . . Nurses noted more than 50 verbal (24.3%) and physical (7.3%) patient/visitor violence incidents over their careers." (Speroni, Fitch, Dawson, Dugan, & Atherton, 2014)

An example of physician abuse of nursing personnel that might have resulted in medical error is provided to illustrate the potential for harm when things go wrong:

****

". . . My patient, a middle-aged man scheduled for a stem-cell transplant, was having textbook symptoms of a heart attack. Serious cardiac side effects can result from the chemical used to preserve stem cells, making the transplant risky if a patient is unstable. An EKG was done, and we were waiting for a cardiologist when the oncology team came by on morning rounds.

"The attending physician heard about the patient's chest pain, then glanced at the EKG while checking his smartphone. 'This does not concern me,' he said, tapping at his screen as he pushed the EKG paper aside.

"This particular doctor was known for his explosive impatience. On a good day his temper simmered just below the surface. On a bad day, he openly seethed. If I asked him to delay the transplant it would be ugly for me; if I said nothing, it could be very dangerous for my patient. So I asked for a delay.

"In the hallway, the doctor, in front of the rounding team, his large body twisted down to put his face close to mine, yelled, 'Why?'

This was intimidation, plain and simple. But it was also an example of a doctor's abusing the legal, established hierarchy between doctors and nurses." (Brown, 1363455920 2013)

****

The risk of infections is present in all settings where nurses are employed such as: ". . . nursing homes, institutions for the retarded, prisons, and outpatient facilities, i.e.: dialysis centers, workplace health centers, or community health clinics. In hospitals, high risk areas include pediatric areas, infectious disease wards, emergency rooms, and ambulatory care facilities.

"Hepatitis B (HBV) is the most prevalent work-related infectious disease in the United States. Although blood is the major source of the virus, it may also be present in saliva, semen, and feces.

"Transmission may occur from a percutaneous stick from a contaminated needle or other sharp instrument (the risk of contracting HBV after a stick with a known contaminated needle is 6–30 percent . . . after contaminated blood enters a break in the skin or splatters onto mucous membranes, or upon ingestion." (Practice, Pope, Snyder, & Mood, 1995)

****

"I felt a sharp sting. Looking down, I saw a small scarlet drop emerging from the tip of my left index finger. I had stabbed my finger against the needle I had just used to anesthetize Jean's skin, a needle I still held in my right hand.

"I stared at the tiny red bloom on my fingertip. And for a moment, I felt the floor beneath my feet give way, pulling everything — Jean, my heart, my work, my life — down with it. I stood there paralyzed, staring at the puncture wound on my fingertip and unable to stop the movie playing in my mind's eye." (Parker-Pope, 1242932704 2009)

****

The issue of the death of or damage to a child tends to be a universal critical incident for First Responders of all types. The instinctive inclination to protect children from harm strikes the soul of the first responder on the scene. Incidents involving children tend to become permanent memories within the minds of those who are dedicated to assist others. The following material details the interaction of EMS personnel as well as ER staff in the identification of an abused child.

****

"EMS is called to the residence of a 2-month-old child who's lethargic and hasn't eaten well for several days... During your assessment, you notice the child isn't acting age appropriate. Initial vital signs after placing the patient in the ambulance reveal: blood pressure 82/46, pulse 146 bpm, respirations 32 and a blood-glucose level of 134 mg/dL. Further assessment reveals bruising to the pinna of the right ear.

"On arrival at the emergency department (ED), the child begins to have periods of apnea, and the hospital healthcare providers intubate the patient. A post-intubation chest X-ray reveals multiple acute and sub-acute rib fractures. The ED staff exposed the patient during their assessment and noted bruising to the left ear and the jaw. There's also bruising found in different stages of healing to the anterior and posterior chest wall.

"The ED staff suspects this patient is a victim of child maltreatment, so the proper authorities are notified. During the investigation, the mother admits to abusing the child (By, n.d.-a)."

****

In the past, many abused or neglected children were missed initially by paramedics and then by nursing staff in the ER. . . . The authors of the following study developed a screening checklist for child abuse as well as training sessions for nurses. They report that: "A total of 104,028 children aged 18 years or younger were included. The screening rate increased from 20% in February 2008 to 67% in December 2009. Significant trend changes were observed after training . . . The detection rate in children screened for child abuse was 5 times higher than that in children not screened." (Louwers et al., 2012)

A final comment on this critical topic is to be found in 2014 statistics from a factsheet that provides information regarding child deaths resulting from abuse or neglect by a parent or a primary caregiver. The authors report that: ". . . nationally estimated 1,580 children died from abuse and neglect in 2014. This translates to a rate of 2.13 children per 100,000 children in the general population and an average of four children dying every day from abuse or neglect.

"Many researchers and practitioners believe that child fatalities due to abuse and neglect are still underreported. One such speculation on national child abuse and neglect deaths in the United States estimates that approximately 50 percent of deaths reported as "unintentional injury deaths" are reclassified after further investigation by medical and forensic experts as deaths due to maltreatment." ("Child Abuse and Neglect Fatalities 2014: Statistics and Interventions - fatality.pdf," 2014)

Major critical incidents forthcoming from manmade circumstances such as terrorist attacks or due to natural disasters such as storms, earth quakes, etc., add further demands and pressures to an often understaffed and highly pressured ER system. Because of these infrequent but highly impactful circumstances, I thought it prudent to discuss a few examples of these unsettling events.

Because of increasing levels of terrorism worldwide, it's wise to look at how nurses cope with this situation in a country where ongoing radical incidents occur with much frequency. The main goal of the following study was to explore the exposure of nurses in Israel to national terror and the levels of distress experienced due to ongoing terror attacks.

Data was collected from 214 nurses from various parts of Israel with the researchers finding that: "... Levels of exposure were associated with burnout, intrusive memories and medium-to high levels of stress." (Ron & Shamai, 2014)."

A classic 1999 study examined the incidence of Post-Traumatic Stress Disorder experienced by rescue workers as a result of a natural disaster. Unfortunately, seventeen years after this article, the same attitude pertaining to the permanency of PTSD symptoms remain among those affected by the experience.

The authors examined stress-specific and general symptomatic distress in emergency services personnel noting that: "A three-group . . . design was used to determine the responses of 322 rescue workers to the Loma Prieta earthquake Interstate 880 Freeway collapse . . . Self-report questionnaires, including measures of incident exposure . . . and emotional distress, and current symptoms, were administered 1.9 years (initial) and 3.5 years (follow-up) after the freeway collapse.

Despite modest symptom improvement at follow-up, rescue workers were at risk for chronic symptomatic distress after critical incident exposure. . . The results suggest that rescue workers, particularly those with more catastrophic exposure and those prone to dissociate at the time of the critical incident, are at risk for chronic symptomatic distress." (Marmar et al., 1999)

Another major concern within the context of stress, burnout and PTSD is the issue of medication addiction among nursing personnel. The authors of the following article note that: "For over 100 years, nurses' particular work conditions have been anecdotally associated with increases in substance abuse. Reasons include job-related stress and easy access to medications. Current research has suggested that the prevalence of nurses with substance use problems is actually similar to, if not less than, that seen in the general population (Monroe, Kenaga, Dietrich, Carter, & Cowan, 2013)."

The authors of the following 2015 articles sent anonymous surveys to 441 active and recent participants of a peer health assistance program. Responses were received from 302 nurses (69%) with the authors noting that: "Nearly half (48%) reported drug or alcohol use at work, and two fifths (40%) felt that their competency level was affected by their use. More than two thirds of respondents thought their problem could have been recognized earlier. The most highly rated barriers to seeking assistance for substance use and mental illness included fear and embarrassment and concerns about losing one's nursing license." (Cares, Pace, Denious, & Crane, 2015)

****

". . . I was able to have a nurse witness a waste with me, and then in turn pocket the excess medication instead of disposing of it. . . I told myself that I would only do it for oral medications and never for an injectable.

. . . Before long, the Percocet was no longer giving me the feeling that it had initially. . . so I started doing the same for all oral opioid analgesics that I could, including codeine and morphine. . . I deluded myself into thinking that injecting morphine intramuscularly or subcutaneously really was not that bad..

. . . I required higher doses to attempt to achieve the same effect. . . When I was not able to use opioids, I began feeling ill, tired, and unfocused; my body started cramping and I was not able to function. . . The day finally came when I was called into my manager's office and I was informed that I had been flagged on the narcotics report. . . .

> Even though I knew the truth of my addiction, I was not ready to admit it to myself or anyone else. Instead, I did what I had been doing since the beginning—I Lied. I had an excuse for almost every opioid with-drawal but they were not believed.
> . . I was terminated from my job. And, I was reported to the state board of nursing for narcotic diversion." (Doe, 2012)

****

Unfortunately, current treatment interventions including Critical Incident Stress Debriefings, "Gold Standard" interventions, medication interventions, etc., do not adequately address the life-altering consequences of frequent exposure to trauma. In my opinion, available treatments for addictive disorders fall within the same category.

As noted earlier, trauma doesn't differentiate between man-made disasters or natural ones. Clara Barton appropriately advised us to disregard precedent, and to have faith in the "possibility of something better." That something is available now in the form of RESET Therapy as well as in other emerging therapies based on neuroscientific knowledge.

Summary:

It is clear that the Affordable Care Act has placed immense pressure on Emergency departments across the country. The intent of the act was to focus on improving access and quality of care to the uninsured. Unfortunately, because of increased demand, many ED systems can no longer handle snowballing needs, thereby producing long delays for admitted patients and increasing levels of pressure on attending staff.

Taking this overview, a step further, administrative pressure to address the increased demand is producing burnout in ER staff with a resulting escalation in medical errors. Ultimately, patient care is likely to deteriorate in these conditions. Examples of the stress forthcoming from a normal 12-hour shift were provided, as exemplified in the varied stories included in the chapter.

While demand for nurses is increasing, the stress associated with the work load is leading to early ending of careers, burnout and ultimately, PTSD. Additionally, abuse of medication, simply because it is readily available in ER settings, becomes another matter of concern.

Examples of Critical Incidents were provided, which were cited by nurses as being primary contributors to their difficulties within the ER setting. A term new to me (boarding) was discussed. This practice often results in a number of problems, including ambulance refusals, prolonged patient waiting times, and increased suffering for those who wait, lying on gurneys in emergency department corridors for hours, and even days, which affects not only their care and comfort but also the primary work of the emergency department staff taking care of emergency department patients." ("Definition of Boarded Patient // ACEP," 2011)

Reference List:

!2013-3rded-advocacyhandbook-interactive.pdf. https://www.emra.org/uploadedfiles/emra/emra_publications/books/!2013-3rded-advocacyhandbook-interactive.pdf

A Day in the Life of an Emergency Room Nurse. http://www.nursetogether.com/day-life-emergency-room-nurse

A stressed-out ER nurse tells her story. (2013, February 8). https://philebersole.wordpress. /2013/02/08/a-stressed-out-er-nurse-tells-her-story/

Brown, T. (1363455920). Healing the Hospital Hierarchy. http://opinionator.blogs.nytimes.com/2013/03/16/healing-the-hospital-hierarchy/

By, B. T. Y. EMS Providers Can Identify Child Abuse. http://www.jems.com/articles /print/volume-

36/issue-10/patient-care/ems-providers-can-identify-child-abuse.html

Cardiac Arrest Statistics. http://cpr.heart.org/ AHAECC /CPRAndECC/General/UCM_477263_Cardiac-Arrest-Statistics.jsp

Cares, A., Pace, E., Denious, J., & Crane, L. A. (2015). Substance use and mental illness among nurses: workplace warning signs and barriers to seeking assistance. *Substance Abuse*, *36*(1), 59–66. https://doi.org/10.1080 /08897077.2014.933725

Child Abuse and Neglect Fatalities 2014: Statistics and Interventions - fatality.pdf. https://www.childwelfare.gov/pubPDFs/fatality.pdf

Definition of Boarded Patient // ACEP. https://www.acep.org/Clinical---Practice-Management/Definition-of-Boarded-Patient-21474 69010/

Doe, J. (2012). My Story: How one Percocet Prescription Triggered my Addiction. *Journal of Medical Toxicology*, *8*(4), 327–330. https://doi.org/10.1007/s13181-012-0268-5

Duarte, J., Pinto-Gouveia, J., & Cruz, B. (2016). Relationships between nurses' empathy, self-compassion and dimensions of professional quality of life: A cross-sectional study. *International Journal of Nursing Studies*, *60*, 1–11. https://doi. org/10.1016/j.ijnurstu .2016 .02.015

Emergency Nurse. https://www.discovernursing.com/specialty/emergency-nurse

Emergency Nursesâ•Ž Experiences with Critical Incidents: A Dissertation - viewcontent.cgi. http://escholarship.umassmed.edu/cgi/viewcontent.cgi?article=1012&context=gsn_diss

FINAL REPORT Suicides by clinicians involved in SIs in the NHS.pdf. http://www.cln.nhs.uk/userfiles/file/FINAL%20REPORT%20Suicides%20by%20clinicians%20involved%20%20in%20SIs%20in%20the%20NHS.pdf

Hidden Grief and Lasting Emotions in Emergency Department Nurses: Ingenta Connect. http://www.ingentaconnect.com/contentone/springer/crnu/2016/00000022/00000004/art00006

http://nursejournal.org, 2017 NurseJournal org |. Registered Nurse Salary & Career Outlook. http://nursejournal.org/registered-nursing/rn-careers-salary-outlook/
https://www.aamc.org/download/100598/data/. https://www.aamc.org/download /100598/data/

I Am One of the Lucky Ones: A Mother's Story of Medical Error. http://www.everydayhealth.com/columns/my-health-story/lucky-ones-mothers-story-medical-error/

Lofton, K. Emergency Medical Workers "Pause" After Traumatic Death. http://wmra.org/post/emergency-medical-workers-pause-after-traumatic-death

Louwers, E. C. F. M., Korfage, I. J., Affourtit, M. J., Scheewe, D. J. H., van de Merwe, M. H., Vooijs-Moulaert, A.-F. S. R., ... de Koning, H. J. (2012). Effects of systematic screening and detection of child abuse in emergency depart ments. *Pediatrics*, *130*(3), 457–464. https://doi.org/10.1542/peds.2011-3527

Marmar, C. R., Weiss, D. S., Metzler, T. J., Delucchi, K. L., Best, S. R., & Wentworth, K. A. (1999). Longitudinal course and predictors of continuing distress following critical incident exposure in emergency services personnel. *The Journal of Nervous and Mental Disease*, *187*(1), 15–22.

Monroe, T. B., Kenaga, H., Dietrich, M. S., Carter, M. A., & Cowan, R. L. (2013). The prevalence of employed nurses identified or enrolled in substance use monitoring programs. *Nursing Research*, *62*(1), 10–15. https://doi.org/10.1097/NNR.0b013e31826ba3ca

msnbc.com, J. A. H. writer. (2011, June 27). Nurse's suicide highlights twin tragedies of medical errors. http://www.nbcnews.com /id/43 529641 /ns/health-health_care/t/ nurses-suicide-highl ights-twin-tragedies-medical-errors/

Parker-Pope, T. (1242932704). When Patients Put Doctors at Risk. http://well.blogs.nytimes com/ 2009/05/21/when-patients-put-doctors-at-risk/

Practice, I. of M. (US) C. on E. E. H. C. in N., Pope, A. M., Snyder, M. A., & Mood, L. H. (1995). *Environmental Hazards for the Nurse as a Worker*. National Academies Press (US).

https://www.ncbi.nlm.nih. gov/books/NBK 232400/

recentworkforcestudiesnov09.pdf. https://report.nih. gov/investigators_and_trainees/acd_bwf/pdf/rec entworkforcestudiesnov09.pdf

Robinson, R., & Stinson, C. K. (2016). Moral Distress: A Qualitative Study of Emergency Nurses. *Dimensions of Critical Care Nursing: DCCN*, *35*(4), 235–240. https://doi.org /10.1097/DCC .0000000 000000185

Ron, P., & Shamai, M. (2014). The impact of ongoing national terror on the community of hospital nurses in Israel. *Community Mental Health Journal*, *50*(3), 354–361. https:// doi.org/10. 1007/s10597-013-9645-z

Shrtstormtrooper. (2014, May 14). ER Nurse Insanity: The Texas Years: Burnout. http://themountains arecalling.blogspot.com/2014/05/burnout.html

Speroni, K. G., Fitch, T., Dawson, E., Dugan, L., & Atherton, M. (2014). Incidence and cost of nurse workplace violence perpetrated by hospital patients or patient visitors. *Journal of Emergency Nursing: JEN: Official Public-ation of the Emergency Department Nurses Association*, *40*(3), 218–228; quiz 295. https://doi.org/10.1016 /j.jen.2013.05.014

Support - National Women's History Museum - NWHM . https://www.nwhm.org/blog/the-evolution-of-nursing/

Wang, S., Liu, Y., & Wang, L. (2015). Nurse burnout: personal and environmental factors as predictors. *International Journal of Nursing Practice*, *21*(1), 78–86. https://doi.org/10.1111/ijn.12216

Chapter Six

ER Physician

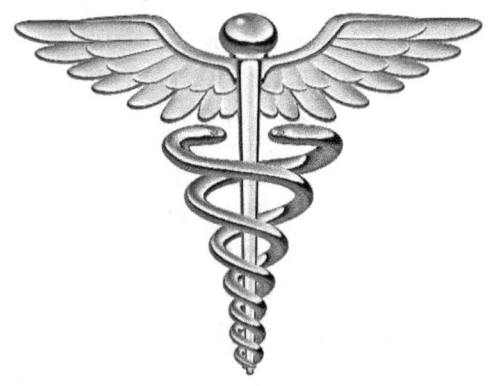

"The physician must be able to tell the antecedents, know the present, and foretell the future — must mediate these things, and have two special objects in view with regard to disease, namely, to do good or to do no harm."

<u>Hippocrates</u>

It is appropriate to briefly discuss the fascinating history of the creation of emergency services in modern times. Although there are earlier reports of systemized attempts to aid others (in 623, Pope Gregory had a hospital built to treat sick, poor or injured Christian pilgrims in Jerusalem), Napoleon Bonaparte's appointment of Dominique Jean Larrey as chief surgeon to his troops marks the initiation of an attempt to save lives on the battlefield.

The authors of the following article note that: "At the time, battlefield medics failed to save many soldiers because the ambulances at the time wouldn't allow them to get near wounded soldiers until fighting ceased, so Larrey developed a 'flying ambulance' which utilized the power of the horse and a four wheeled wagon. This new vehicle was capable of taking wounded soldiers to get emergency care much quicker." ("A BRIEF HISTORY OF EMERGENCY MEDICAL SERVICES | Badge & Wallet," 2015)

The onset of the emergency room concept was slow in coming to the US as reported in the following article: ". . . The original 'Accident Room' at Johns Hopkins Hospital was a two-bed facility, and the first patients were treated free of charge. A police patrol wagon transported patients because ambulance services were not yet widely available.

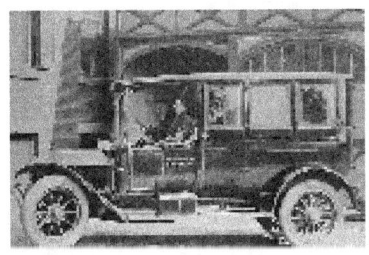

In the 1950s, Hopkins physicians originated the Emergency Squad Doctor Plan so that a physician on call could be taken to the scene of an accident to administer on-the-spot treatment." (Molnar, n.d.)

". . . In 1960, there was no emergency medicine as a defined academic specialty. Typical hospital emergency rooms staffing patterns used resident, intern, other hospital staff physicians, or rotating on-call duty of all specialties including those such as psychiatry and even pathology. . . At least half of all ambulance services 'were' run by morticians or funeral directors because they had vehicles that could transport people horizontally, often using untrained staff. There were no national coordinating organizations.

". . . Before the establishment of emergency medicine in the U.S., emergencies that needed a specific specialist not in attendance were given to whatever physician could be found, regardless of expertise. Often this was a very junior doctor in training. While some older specialists still refer to these as 'the good old days'. Unfortunately, they were not good for patients who had emergencies at the 'wrong time'...

"The problems with this approach were twofold. First, even (in) the largest hospitals all specialists may not be available in the light of a typical day, but without the specialty of emergency medicine it is rarely possible to provide specialist care at 3 a.m. or on a holiday. Second, and more fundamental, is that atypical presentations of disease often make it unclear which specialist the patient needs in a timely manner." (Suter, 2012)

We have come a long way since the "flying ambulance" yet it appears that we still have miles to go in the development of ER services. Conflicts between administrative requirements and governmental regulations, as opposed to the provision of quality care, add undue stress to an often-overburdened system. Furthermore, the push for increasing levels of patient satisfaction scores challenges the physician and ER staff to at times compromise what they consider to be best practice procedures.

As the traditional first recipient of those requiring emergency intervention within a hospital setting, the ER system is a crucial component of the first responder system. When operating smoothly and efficiently, team building ensues across all professionals involved in the service. However, when chronically overloaded, stress becomes a prominent theme that permeates the staff at all levels leading to burnout, compassion fatigue and ultimately, PTSD.

The structure/framework for this chapter will vary somewhat from other chapters due to the prolonged educational requirements of the physician. We will begin with the job description and job tempo, then proceed to describe stress aspects of the physician educational experience including: pre-med; medical; internship; residency/specialty training. As utilized in prior chapters, the following components will also be discussed: family stress impact; special incidents; medical errors; stress effects and their association with PTSD; physician medication abuse; physician suicide.

The end goal of engagement of training in the medical field is to become licensed to practice medicine. "Licensure, which is mandatory, is earned by passing a national qualification exam generally after completion of medical school. Board certification demonstrates that a physician has met the minimum requirements to practice medicine by establishing expertise." ("ER Doctor Requirements, " n.d.)

". . . Over half of EM physicians (55%) have seen an influx of patients' due to the Affordable Care

Act (ACA)... Among those who said quality had worsened, 21% had a higher patient load and 18% reported no increase... Just over two thirds (67%) of EM physicians spend 30-45 hours per week seeing patients, and only 19% spend more than that.

"... Bureaucratic tasks were the prime cause of physician burnout, according to this year's Medscape Lifestyle Report (and in previous ones as well). Second was spending too many hours at work. Among EM physicians responding to this year's survey, 41% of those who are self-employed and 49% of their employed peers spend 10 hours or more per week on paperwork and administrative tasks." (Kane & Peckham, 2015)

In regard to future employment opportunity, "the U.S. Bureau of Labor Statistics predicted an overall 14% increase in employment of physicians and surgeons over the 2014-2024 decade. The aging baby boomer population is part of the reason for this faster-than-average growth." ("ER Doctor Require-ments," n.d.)

The pace of working in an emergency room setting requires the ability to cope with a variety of situations within the context of an unpredictable pattern. Patient flow is variable, but heightened emotions among those who are sick is a given. For those who are attracted to becoming a physician and like variety and excitement, this would be a good occupational choice.

Night shift tends to involve more traumas such as gun shots and stabbings. Day shift is inclined to involve more team work and supportive interaction among varied hospital staff.

****

"... I think I am a typical emergency medicine physician. I care. I don't EVER want to make a mistake. I don't want to miss anything. I don't want my patients to be unhappy. I don't want to let administration down. I want answers, solutions and nice neat boxes of 'all better.' ...

"So, why do emergency physicians burn out? Let me give you my theory... We all care about meeting core measures, accomplishing department goals, doing a great job, making people well and happy, serving as team leaders and, ultimately, providing the best medical care possible based on current evidences.

"... We hold it together to mechanically and precisely insert complicated intravenous lines, perform and interpret ultrasounds, and order medications on crashing patients. We beam when we are able to tell the "infertile" couple in Room 7 they will be expecting twins. Moments later we dodge the arm of the knife-wielding, crazed, homeless man who is losing his battles with liver failure and bedbugs.

"Welcome to life in the real ER.

". . . I have gone to the bathroom to breathe, pray, and secure the door on the memories of painful patient encounters: the heart attacks at the ballfield; the toddler falling over the stair railing; the joy-ride meets tree; the drugged-out mom with the malnourished infant; the international traveler (coding, gasping, hypoxic) from a pulmonary embolism; the suicides; the gang violence; the end-of-life goodbyes; and the many, many overdoses.

. . . I could go on detailing why I am scorched (maybe not burned yet), making a list as long as the causes of tachycardia, but I won't. I think I am done." ("In My Shoes: Facing burnout as emergency medicine physician | In My Shoes | richmond.com," 2016)

****

The path to becoming a physician is replete with challenge and stress from the application process building throughout the many and varied educational aspects as described below:

"Within the pre-med experience, there is concern about increasing levels of stress during undergraduate medical training. The authors of the following study explored the presence of perceived stress among undergraduate medical students. A 10-item questionnaire was used to assess academic sources of stress and their severity. "The overall mean perceived stress score was 29.58 . . . and 46.3% of the participants were in the group of more stressed. (Chowdhury et al., 2017)

****

"I am almost 26 years old, I spent 5 years doing undergraduate work, I will be nearly 35 years old before I can ever see a patient as an attending physician, and I will be in debt over a quarter of a million dollars. As it stands now, we will almost certainly have some sort of universal health care that will no doubt bring physician salaries down, and just last year the government changed the way our student loans could be paid back letting interest gain while we are still in training.

Couple that with a public that sees us as glorified car mechanics that they can sue when things go wrong, an aging population that wants 'everything done' to keep them alive even if they have no idea who or what they even are, and a payment system that gives dermatologists more money and more time off than family doctors, the future looks less than bright.

"Oh, and did I mention that every student in medical school wants to be either a dermatologist, plastic surgeon, or an orthopedic surgeon, thus creating the most competitive hostile environment. At my school people routinely misplace books in the library so others won't find them." (Parker-Pope, 1225378222 2008)

****

The completion of pre-med requirements takes the student into the next level of driven engagement with others who are striving to succeed in an ever-increasing world of competitive involvement. It seems as though one advances to a greater level of stress with each accomplishment. Is it any wonder that so many of our ER physicians complain of stress by the time they finally complete the ordeal of medical training. The following article details some of the aspects of this challenging process.

"At the outset of education, a medical school student must overcome the stress of the interview. Then there are exams and apprenticeships. To top it all there is contact with lecturers, students and other academic staff. Summing up all these factors, a medical student during the educational process is subjected to constant stress, which she/he must overcome. It is worth noting that not every person (student) is able to cope with this pressure, and that negative life events in this context can confer risk of depression and suicidal thinking.

"Next, the candidate faces the process of application to a medical school setting. Applicants who have completed prerequisite coursework, have earned a high GPA, can produce strong letters of recommendation and have achieved outstanding MCAT (Medical College Admissions Test) scores have a fighting chance of getting into a respected medical school." (Kane & Peckham, 2015)

"Based on a cross-sectional self-reported survey, medical students perceive that exams are the most common source of chronic stress for young people entering adulthood... The study shows that chronic exposure to stressful conditions may lead to psychological discomfort, mental health problems, depression and anxiety symptoms which might increase risk for suicidal thinking.

"Additionally, it has been noted that stress contributes to exacerbation of viral and infectious diseases and allergies in the researched group. Students are aware of the need to combat stress and suicidal thinking and of the fact that it can protect them against the development of illnesses such as depression and other mental ailments." (Rosiek, Rosiek-Kryszewska, Leksowski, & Leksowski, 2016)

". . . During the co-called 'practical year' (PJ), which completes the degree course, a striking 20% of medical students have been shown to reach values in the Maslach Burnout Inventory (MBI) indicating elevated burnout risk." (*Die Wahrheit über Burnout - Stress am Arbeitsplatz und was | Christina Maslach | Springer*, 2001)

"Maslach et al. were able to show that these are accompanied by emotional exhaustion, increasing depersonalization and feelings of reduced personal accomplishment. ("The Maslach Burnout Inventory Manual,") They further defined the experience of contact as emotionally overwhelming and the loss of the ability to regenerate as emotional exhaustion. Depersonalization means that physicians have negative, cynical attitudes and impersonal feelings toward their patients. Hence, Maslach et al. often refer to this diagnostic dimension as 'cynicism'. The feeling of reduced personal accomplishment refers to the tendency to experience one's own activity as insufficiently competent and/or effective." (Bugaj et al., 2016)

****

"It did not take long for my excitement to wane. Within only a few days of starting my residency, I was called "retarded" and referred to with homophobic slurs. Women were commonly referred to with misogynistic labels. I was given no organized instruction on how to perform my duties, only criticized because I didn't do things as the supervisor I'd had the prior day had taught me.

"My first month of residency was the worst experience of my entire adult education. I think anyone who has borne witness to television shows that depict medical education can appreciate that doctors can be hard on you as a trainee, but the extent at which personal attacks were levied at myself and other professionals is something that I didn't anticipate and never came close to witnessing as a medical student. I was assured that this happens everywhere, but to this day, I refuse to accept that standard." ("A tragic physician story the match doesn't want you to hear about," 2015)

****

". . . Rotations through all the departments in a hospital begin in the third year, which provide the needed experience that allows medical students to select an area of specialization for their residency.

"Matching is the term used for the process . . . for finding a placement in a paid post-graduate residency program in which a Doctor of Medicine (MD) becomes an ER doctor. Some ER residencies require that residents serve a preliminary year in a less hectic medical environment and gradually acquire the confidence and skills necessary to work in the ER.

****

"My resident told me today that he was planning on giving antibiotics to a kid with a fever. I asked him where the fever was coming from - he said he didn't see anything on the exam, but the parents were pretty insistent that the kid needed antibiotics, and he was tired of arguing. 'Plus,' he added, 'it's good for patient satisfaction scores.'

". . . I popped into the room and saw a happy, healthy, smiling 5 year old pulling all the paper towels from the dispenser. He ran over to the door, gave me a high-five/low-five/fist bump combo, and then asked me when he was able to go home and watch cartoons. I did an exam which revealed absolutely nothing abnormal.

". . . 'But he's got a fever,' she said, 'every time he has a fever my pediatrician puts him on antibiotics. My child *needs* antibiotics!' Over the years, I've gotten very good at having this conversation with parents. Usually they leave the ER happy and reassured that their child looks healthy and well, with the understanding that antibiotics will make no difference - and in fact, may cause harm, predisposing their child to vomiting, diarrhea, allergic reactions, and resistant bacterial infections. In this case, mom was having none of it. There was no way she was leaving happy without antibiotics. And so, in the end, she left - but unhappy, and without antibiotics." ("Agraphia," 2005)

****

It is expected that an emergency room will experience periods of intense demand. An example of the building pace of an ER physician is provided in the following report: "Daily work starts rather slowly at our department... However time flies, the ED beds are used (and re-used), the *fast-track* treating minor casualties gets really busy and you work at a faster pace; maybe you decide to skip lunch today.

"Suddenly you realize patients don't move to the wards anymore, since the admitted patients are still occupying the beds... Nurses get stressed because there are insufficient trolleys so ambulance crews have to wait for a vacant bed or trolley; you wonder if it would be wise to *diverse the ambulances* to another hospital.

"In the mean while the *triage* nurse decides to use the fast track beds for some very sick patients, since she prioritizes incoming patients according to their emergency... You end up with a waiting room full of patients with minor illnesses or trauma waiting for treatment...

"You realize *patient satisfaction* will be low whenever waiting times get longer. Some patients decide to try out another hospital and leave against medical advice or even *leave before being seen* by a doctor.

"At the end of the day you start to discuss the remaining patients under your care to the colleague taking over; seems quite a few patients are still in the department waiting for a surgical *specialist advice* which you requested a few hours ago." ("Working as an Emergency Physician," 2015)

****

"He was a 50-something, shabbily dressed guy in somewhat of a constant state of disrepair. There was a musty odor of tobacco about him, and when the nurse entered the room he sneered 'Oh, there you are. So there IS someone actually attending patient needs today. Get me a damn soda, I'm thirsty.' He had been triaged, registered, and taken to a room within 25 minutes of arrival. His wife piped in, 'Make it a Coke for him and a Mountain Dew for me. We don't do Diet.'

"I walked in the room to a hostile environment... He had his arms crossed and began to lay into me before I could say a word. 'I want an MRI. I hurt my back lifting something a couple hours ago, I've had a bulging disk before, and I've been waiting now for the better part of 30 minutes to see ANYBODY who is competent around here.'

"I took a mental breath, calmed the raging inner demons, and introduced myself. I apologized for not seeing him earlier as I had been performing CPR in another room and broke away just as soon as I was free.

"I'll cut the story short here and get to the chase. He left the ER with a diagnosis of back sprain *sans* MRI, shouting at staff, extremely angry...but it was clear from our first interaction that this was inevitable. Interestingly, he didn't come to the ER for pain control - he came because he wanted an MRI, and was livid that I wouldn't give him what he wanted." ("Agraphia," 2005)

****

Within this stressful environment, it is anticipated that cumulative exposure to trauma will ultimately produce burnout in attending staff, including physicians. Within this context, a 2016 report defines burnout as: ". . . loss of enthusiasm for work, feelings of cynicism, and a low sense of personal accomplishment. In this year's *Medscape* report, the highest percentages of burnout occurred in critical care, urology, and emergency medicine, all at 55%. . . Of note, however, burnout rates for all specialties are higher this year than in 2015.

"A survey published in the *Mayo Clinic Proceedings* compared burnout between 2011 and 2014 and observed an increase in the percentage of physicians reporting at least one burnout symptom from 45.5% to 54.4%." ("Medscape Lifestyle Report 2016: Bias and Burnout," 2016)

There is little question that the practice of medicine can be demanding and stressful. Indeed, numerous studies have found (Anderson Spickard, Gabbe, & Christensen, 2002) (Shanafelt et al., 2009) that many physicians have experienced: "professional burnout, a syndrome characterized by a loss of enthusiasm for work (emotional exhaustion), feelings of cynicism (depersonalization), and a low sense of personal accomplishment. These findings suggest that burnout may: "erode professionalism, influence quality of care, increase the risk for medical errors, and promote early retirement.

"Burnout also seems to have adverse personal consequences for physicians, including contributions to broken relationships, problematic alcohol use, and suicidal ideation." (Shanafelt et al., 2012)

Within the context of relationships, I will next explore family dynamics among those physicians who specialize in emergency medicine. Divorce among physicians in general is no more common than in other healthcare professions and non-healthcare professions as noted in the following article:

"In fact, the prevalence and incidence of divorce among physicians were similar to pharmacists and dentists and substantially lower than that of nurses, healthcare executives, lawyers, and other non-healthcare professionals. Despite evidence that professional obligations among physicians, including long and sometimes unpredictable work hours, may conflict with personal and family life, we found no evidence that divorce among physicians was more common as a result.

Secondly, female physicians were substantially more likely to be divorced than male physicians. Hours worked per week were positively correlated with divorce only for female physicians and not for male physicians, suggesting that differences in divorce rates between male and female physicians may be partly attributable to differential responses of divorce to hours worked." ("Divorce among physicians and other healthcare professionals in the United States: analysis of census survey data | The BMJ," 2016)

****

"I quit medicine. I was five months out of residency, and I was leaving medicine. I had dedicated my heart, soul, several years of my life along with weekends, holidays, special events, and my children's first words to this honorable profession. Medicine was never suppose to "just be" my job. It was suppose to be my calling, and it had betrayed me.

"Not only did I leave the office night after night completely frustrated, hopeless and exhausted, I showed up each morning in the same state, if not slightly worse. The personal accomplishment of healing was gone. The enthusiasm of service, gone. The love of human kind, gone.

"I was drained, sucked dry and running on empty. I had developed physical symptoms: myalgias, headaches, IBS, palpitations, anxiety. But, honestly, the scariest part, I quit caring. It just became about ending the day, finishing one more chart, seeing one more now so at least it was one less tomorrow. No amount of incentives were going to bring me back or cure me." (Weisman, 2016)

****

When a person loses enthusiasm for what was previously a primary drive and hasn't replaced it with another focus, it is likely that a burnout process has advanced to the stage of compassion fatigue. When this occurs, medical errors are more likely to occur. One recent study found that: "where a lack of teamwork (i.e. poor communication, lack of team structure, lack of cross-monitoring) was implicated in a particular incident of ED medical error, an average of 8.8 teamwork failures occurred per case [and] more than half of the deaths and permanent disabilities that occurred were judged avoidable.

"Unfortunately, certain cultural (i.e. "a focus on the errors of others and a 'blame-and-shame' culture") and structural (i.e. lack of standardization and equipment incompatibilities) aspects of emergency medicine often result in a lack of disclosure of medical error and near misses to patients and other caregivers.

"While concerns about malpractice liability is one reason why disclosure of medical errors is not made, some have noted that disclosing the error and providing an apology can mitigate malpractice risk.

Ethicists uniformly agree that the disclosure of a medical error that causes harm is the duty of a care provider.

"The key components of disclosure include "honesty, explanation, empathy, apology, and the chance to lessen the chance of future errors. . . The nature of emergency medicine is such that error will likely always be a substantial risk of emergency care." ("Emergency medicine," 2016)

While the above material provides error rates and averages, the following article personalizes the effects of making an error when caring for others. The author notes that: "We tend to avoid our everyday stories of insecurity, frustration, and minor irritations. We keep quiet about the shameful bits—forgotten dosages, missed intubations, lost arguments against consultants. We do not talk about second-guessing our career path, missing important deadlines, our rising cholesterol, or an impending divorce.

"Perhaps not surprisingly then, emergency physicians suffer from some of the highest rates of burnout compared to other physicians. A 2012 survey across multiple medical specialties in the U.S. found that up to 60% of practicing emergency medicine physicians admit to feelings of burnout. Furthermore, as many as 75% of residents meet criteria for burnout in some studies." (Chung & MD, 2016)

"It is well known that communication deficits are among the most important causes for critical incidents . . . Information processing in emergency situations is specifically difficult, because there are several challenging issues: 1) time pressure; 2) team with multiple members involved; 3) high distraction probability; 4) several handovers possible; 5) high degree of non-verbal communication (action performing communication like performing procedures); and 6) limited resources for documentation.

"We found that 27.5% of all reported incidents were related to communication deficits. . . It is striking that in many reports team members, mostly paramedics, complain that advice was not followed by other team members, mostly physicians. . . Disregarding advice leads to frustration, which can have a negative effect on future situations if not discussed after finishing the case. Team discussion and debriefing are part of training scenarios and current guidelines recommend this. . . We consider an explanation to the team for certain decisions as well as a short discussion about the case afterwards is important to improve team work.

". . . Lacking or wrong labelling of medication can lead to medication error with sometimes disastrous results. . . The double check or four-eye-principle means that two persons have to confirm the correct drug and dose prior to drug administration in addition to other safety methods." (Hohenstein et al., 2016)

The earlier described environment related to medical errors as well as compassion fatigue also fosters a tendency to seek self-medication alternatives as a means of coping with internal distress. The following article found that: "Approximately 10% to 12% of physicians will develop a substance use disorder during their careers, a rate similar to or exceeding that of the general population.

"Although physicians' elevated social status brings many tangible and intangible rewards, it also has an isolating effect when they are confronted with a disease such as addiction, which has a social stigma. This isolation can lead to disastrous consequences, both in delaying the recognition of and in intervening in the disease process, as well as in the attendant risk of death by inadvertent overdose or suicide." (Berge, Seppala, & Schipper, 2009)

The cumulative effects of stress lead to despondency, isolation and depression. The following author suggests that: ". . . because of the stigma associated with depression in almost all cultures, which seems to be greatly magnified among medical practitioners, self-reporting likely underestimates the prevalence of the disease in medical populations. . .

"With an increasing tendency to self-isolate, self-destructive tendencies emerge leading to suicidal ideation. A 2016 article on this topic suggests that: "It has been known for more than 150 years that physicians have an increased propensity to die by suicide. It was estimated in 1977 that on average the United States loses the equivalent of at least one small medical school or a large medical school class to suicide. Exact numbers are not known. Although it is impossible to estimate with accuracy because of inaccurate cause of death reporting and coding, the number most often used is approximately 3-400 physicians/year, or perhaps a doctor a day.

"Of all occupations and professions, the medical profession consistently hovers near the top of occupations with the highest risk of death by suicide. . . Perhaps even more alarming is that, after accidents, suicide is the most common cause of death among medical students." ("Physician Suicide," 2016)

Summary

A primary criterion for successfully completing the ordeal of becoming a physician appears to be the successful management of increasing levels of stress. Apparently, those who can survive this process can become doctors. In those who can't, what becomes of them? I assume that those who start the process are among the most intellectually gifted among us. Might there be a better way to harness this potential?

Now if it could be demonstrated to me that this 'baptism by fire' is a crucial and necessary component in the provision of quality health care, I might give my perspective a second thought. Alternatively, it seems like a sure way to dehumanize the intended primary provider of health care. Terms such as depersonalization, cynicism, professional burnout, isolating effect, etc., permeate the stress related literature pertaining to emergency room care. Is this truly the way to honor the Hippocrates mandate: "to do good or to do no harm"?

The increased quantity of mandated paperwork is clearly another negative contributing factor to burnout among those providing ER services. In our computer savvy age, isn't it feasible to modify and reduce governmental and administrative requirements related to documentation of provided services? In the same vein, a primary complaint by the ER service provider is the distorted expectations of the clientele using the service. Is patient satisfaction in the ER setting really to be a primary driver in the provision of care?

Medical errors clearly seem to be associated with communication deficits. A team strategy with use of the four-eye-principle surely seems like a logical means to reduce unnecessary mistakes of this kind. But has the ER doctor or involved specialists been taught to function as a member of a team?

Finally, the cumulative effects of stress and exposure to trauma wreaks havoc on the health and wellness of the exposed individual. Can we really afford to lose one skilled doctor per day through suicide? The same can be said for those involved in the training process for becoming a doctor. Given that the medical field in general is a product of a multifactorial product, mightn't an intervention that can neutralize the cumulative effects of stress be of some value within the ER setting? Indeed, wouldn't alternative interventions that can minimize the cumulative effects of stress be of interest to those who function in high stress occupations. I believe that maintaining the quality of life of those who are there 24/7 to assist us is certainly an objective worth pursuing.

References

A BRIEF HISTORY OF EMERGENCY MED-ICAL SERVICES | Badge & Wallet. (2015, April 1). https://www.badgeandwallet.com/ news /brief-history-emergency-medical-services

A tragic physician story the match doesn't want you to hear about. http://www.kevinmd.com /blog/2015/01/tragic-physician-story-match-doesnt-want-hear.html

Agraphia. http://www.agraphia.net/

Anderson Spickard, J., Gabbe, S. G., & Christensen, J. F. (2002). Mid-Career Burnout in General-ist and Specialist Physicians. *JAMA*, *288*(12), 1447–1450. https://doi. org/10.1001 /jama.288.12.1447

Berge, K. H., Seppala, M. D., & Schipper, A. M. (2009). Chemical Dependency and the Physician. *Mayo Clinic Proceedings*, *84*(7), 625–631.

Bugaj, T. J., Mücksch, C., Schmid, C., Junne, F., Erschens, R., Herzog, W., & Nikendei, C. (2016). Peer-led Stress Prevention Seminars in the First Year of Medical School – A Project Report. *GMS Journal for Medical Education*, *33*(1). https://doi.org/10.3205 /zma001002

Chowdhury, R., Mukherjee, A., Mitra, K., Naskar, S., Karmakar, P. R., & Lahiri, S. K. (2017). Perceived psychological stress among undergraduate medical students: Role of academic factors. *Indian Journal of Public Health*, *61*(1), 55–57. https://doi.org/10. 4103/0019-557X.200253

Chung, A. S., & MD. (2016, August 26). stories to live by. https://akosmed.com/2016/08/26 /stories-to-live-by/

Die Wahrheit über Burnout - Stress am Arbeitsplatz und was | Christina Maslach | Springer. http: //www.springer.com/de/book/ 9783211835722

Divorce among physicians and other healthcare professionals in the United States: analysis of census survey data | The BMJ. http ://www . bmj.com/content/350/bmj.h706

Emergency medicine. (2016, November 29). In *Wikipedia.* https://en.wikipedia .org/w /index. php?title=Emergency_medicine& oldid=752049416

ER Doctor Requirements: Info for Aspiring Emer-gency Room Doctors. http://study.com /articles/ER_Doctor_Requirements_Info_for_As piring_Emergency_Room_Doctors.html

Hohenstein, C., Fleischmann, T., Rupp, P., Hempel, D., Wilk, S., & Winning, J. (2016). German critical incident reporting system database of prehospital emergency medicine: Analysis of reported communication and medication errors between 2005–2015. *World Journal of Emergency Medicine*, 7(2), 90–96. https ://doi .org/10.5847 /wjem.j.1920-8642.2 016.02.002

In My Shoes: Facing burnout as emergency medicine physician | In My Shoes | richmond.com. http ://www.richmond. com/life/in-my-shoes/in-my-shoes-facing-burnout-as-emergency-medicine-physician /article_28953528-510d-56e6-8ecf-1a5e313cf0ff.html

Kane, L., & Peckham, C. (2015). *Medscape physician compensation report 2014.*

Medscape Lifestyle Report 2016: Bias and Burnout. http://www.medscape.com/features/slideshow/lifestyle/2016/public/overview

Molnar, H. History of the Department of Emergency Medicine. http://www. Hopkinsmedicine.org/emergencymedicine/history/

Parker-Pope, T. (1225378222). The Misery of the Med Student. https://well.blogs.nytimes.com/2008/10/30/the-misery-of-the-med-student/

Physician Suicide: Overview, Depression in Phy-sicians, Problems With Treating Physician Depression. (2016). http://emedicine.medscape.com/article/806779-overview

Rosiek, A., Rosiek-Kryszewska, A., Leksowski, Ł., & Leksowski, K. (2016). Chronic Stress and Suicidal Thinking Among Medical Students. *International Journal of Environmental Research and Public Health, 13*(2). https://doi.org/10.3390/ijerph13020212

Shanafelt, T. D., Balch, C. M., Bechamps, G. J., Russell, T., Dyrbye, L., Satele, D., ... Freischlag, J. A. (2009). Burnout and career satisfaction among American surgeons. *Annals of Surgery, 250*(3), 463–471. https:// doi.org/10.1097/SLA.0b013e3181ac4dfd

Shanafelt, T. D., Boone, S., Tan, L., Dyrbye, L. N., Sotile, W., Satele, D., ... Oreskovich, M. R.

(2012). Burnout and Satisfaction With Work - Life Balance Among US Physicians Relative to the General US Population. *Archives of Internal Medicine*, *172*(18), 1377–1385. https ://doi.org/10.1001 /archinternmed.2012.3199

Suter, R. E. (2012). Emergency medicine in the United States: a systemic review. *World Journal of Emergency Medicine*, *3*(1), 5–10. https://doi.org/10.5847/wjem.j.issn.1920-8642.2012.01.001

Chapter Seven

Dispatchers/Telecommunicators

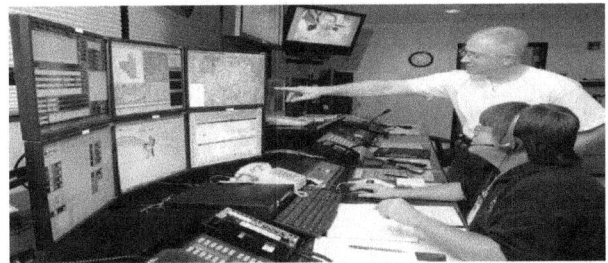

If your eyes could see what my ears have heard, you would weep like me. If your eyes could see what my ears have heard, you would spend countless hours in your bed staring at the ceiling.

If your eyes could see what my ears have heard, then you would cry for the woman who is losing her husband of decades. If your eyes could see what my ears have heard, you would know that gunfire is always near. If your eyes could see what my ears have heard, that house fire would not be so spectacular.

If your eyes could see what my ears have heard, the lost child would be like one of your own. If your eyes could see what my ears have heard, that traffic stop would not be so routine. If your eyes could see what my ears have heard, you would understand.   -
Author Unknown

"Within the United States, there are now more than 6,000 primary and secondary public safety answering points (PSAPs), all of which are staffed by professionals who are highly trained and skilled in emergency communications.

"911 dispatchers are the heartbeat of the nation's 911 system and are the professionals called upon to ensure that citizens receive the best emergency communications and dispatch services by remaining calm, gathering information, and providing assistance to individuals in need.

"Their work involves answering inquiries, referring calls to appropriate law enforcement agencies or emergency medical services companies, determining the response requirements and prioritizing situations, and dispatching units according to a set of established procedures.

"911 dispatcher jobs require excellent communication skills and the ability to work under stressful situations. 911 operators take all applicable information from the caller, including details and the address of the emergency. Through gathering of information, 911 operators are then able to dispatch the appropriate team or transfer the call to the applicable agency. Many 911 dispatchers are also qualified to provide medical information to the caller until emergency help arrives." ("911 Dispatcher Job Description | 911 Operator Job Description," n.d.)

****

"New York City - A shortage of medics and a surge in heat-related 911 calls left the city struggling to respond to medical emergencies last week - and the dangerous situation could worsen as summer intensifies and more FDNY EMS workers jump ship to become fire-fighters, sources told The Post.

"Dozens of ailing people waited more than an hour for a response after dialing 911 last week. During one two-hour period on a sweltering afternoon, six calls were stacked up for more than an hour, and 12 were delayed more than 30 minutes, according to Emergency Medical Service dispatch records reviewed by The Post.

"A shrinking work force strained to respond to a flood of about 15,000 calls over four days - the same amount the city of Boston averages in a month. On a normal working day, the city's 2,000 emergency medical technicians, paramedics and their supervisors get about 3,200 medical calls.

"But last week demand spiked abruptly, going as high as 4,606 during one 24-hour period as temperatures sizzled. Eight people suffered heat-related deaths last week, the city medical examiner said. The sudden surge left dozens of calls queuing in EMS dispatch centers in The Bronx and Brooklyn. An overheated 65-year-old woman with high blood pressure waited nearly two hours for a crew.

"Medics didn't reach a 37-year-old woman suffering from vomiting and stomach pains for an hour and 14 minutes." ("New York City - Critical Shortage Of EMS Workers," 2008)

****

"Although the job description and the job duties of a 911 dispatcher are fairly straightforward, the challenges and rewards of this profession may not always be so evident. Here are the specifics of a 911 dispatcher job that, although may not appear on a job description, are fundamental aspects of this career:

- Emergency dispatching can be incredibly taxing and is therefore not for everyone. No amount of training and education can prepare an individual to handle a frantic caller or a caller whose life is in danger. Some people can be calm in these situations, while others simply cannot. 911 dispatchers must be able to keep their stress at bay and handle their emotions at all times.

- Teamwork is essential to the success of a 911 dispatcher. Professionals in emergency communications must be able rely on each other to get the job done because no one person can do everything at once.

- Multi-tasking is important because 911 dispatchers may be required to keep a caller calm, dispatch emergency services, and provide medical assistance at the same time.

- 911 dispatchers must be able to recover from difficult situations. Although many times these professionals will second guess their actions following particularly difficult calls and feel the burden of these calls, letting work become overwhelming can result in undue anxiety and stress.

- A job in emergency dispatching can be incredibly rewarding, particularly following a situation where emergency communication services help save a life. The sense of gratification and fulfillment experienced following a harrowing 911 call is one of the reasons many of these professionals remain in this field for a long period of time." ("911 Dispatcher Jobs | 911 Operator Jobs," n.d.)

"Most police, fire, and ambulance dispatchers have a high school diploma. Many states require dispatchers to have training and certification. In addition, candidates must pass a written exam and a typing test.

"In some instances, applicants may need to pass a background check, lie detector and drug tests, and tests for hearing and vision. Most states require dispatchers to be U.S. citizens, and some jobs require a driver's license. Experience using computers and in customer service can be helpful. The ability to speak Spanish is also desirable in this occupation.

"The median annual wage for police, fire, and ambulance dispatchers was $38,870 in May 2016... The lowest 10 percent earned less than $25,100, and the highest 10 percent earned more than $61,270. Most dispatchers work 8- to 12-hour shifts, but some agencies require even longer ones. Overtime is common in this occupation. Because emergencies can happen at any time, dispatchers are required to work some shifts on evenings, weekends, and holidays.

"Employment of police, fire, and ambulance dispatchers is projected to decline 3 percent from 2014 to 2024. Although the prevalence of cell phones has increased the number of calls that dispatchers receive, advanced 9-1-1 systems have increased the efficiency of emergency communication centers, allowing them to serve broader regions than before. Consolidation of these centers is expected to reduce the employment of dispatchers.

". . . Overall job prospects should be favorable because the work of a dispatcher remains stressful and demanding, leading some applicants to seek other types of work. The majority of positions will come from the need to replace the large number of dispatchers expected to transfer to other occupations or leave the labor force. Those with good communication skills and experience using computers should have the best job prospects." ("Police, Fire, and Ambulance Dispatchers," n.d.)

****

"When you started your job as a dispatcher, if you were anything like me, Adam Timm, you probably had no idea what to expect. Your visits to the dispatch center to listen to the action and stories from dispatcher friends did little to mentally prepare you for the realities of the job. Even by filling out that checklist on your application.

By filling out this application I have been forewarned that:

___ I may have to work any shift round the clock.

___ I will handle calls of an urgent and life-threatening nature.

___ The people calling me may not be nice.

___ I may not recognize myself in a couple of years.

"... Over time you will learn that your big heart and desire to save the world can expose you to a new challenge: burnout." (Timm & Ph.D, 2015)

****

"... emergency communication specialists (telecommunicators) are considered the gatekeepers for critical emergency information used by police officers, firefighters and paramedics. Emerging technology used by telecommunicators has increased operational efficiency through reduction of emergency response time while simultaneously increasing the number of calls processed per shift.

"Telecommunicators' emotional labor is heightened and agitated by the extreme variations in the caller's emergency circumstance. Telecommunicators are expected to remain emotionally stable regardless of the caller's situation while defusing, decoding and relaying potentially life-saving information to the appropriate authorities. They work in highly structured environments where their performance is regularly monitored and assessed for purposes of improving public safety." (Martin, 2016)

"A group of newly hired 911 dispatchers has begun an intensive training period to prepare them for the realities of answering emergency calls from people in the midst of life's most stressful situations.

"The job requires the dispatchers to bring sound judgment, street savvy, compassion, patience, and, occasionally, a thick skin to every call. Over the course of the 480 hours of training, dispatchers will review protocols for more than 100 types of calls and learn techniques to calm callers and quickly obtain crucial information for first responders.

". . . The Minneapolis 911 center averages about 2,000 calls a day in the summer and about 1,500 calls a day in the winter. The average answer time is 7½ seconds; however, call waiting time varies with the situation. Call answer times can increase on a busy summer night when many people are out.

"Besides the variability of how many incidents occur on any given day, call waiting time can increase significantly when scores or even hundreds of people call 911 about the same issue. A big incident — a bar fight or a car accident, for example — can be witnessed by many people, all of whom can easily make calls with their cell phones."

("Newly hired 911 dispatchers begin training - City of Minneapolis," 2013)

As provided in earlier chapters, the organization of this chapter includes job description and employment parameters. Additionally, I will delineate job tempo, family impact; special incidents; employee burnout; physical and mental stress effects and their association with Compassion Fatigue/PTSD; suicide.

It is now well recognized that vicarious trauma (Perlman & Saakvitne, 1995), also referred to as compassion fatigue, generally describes the cost of caring for others (Figley, 1982). Although the following article refers to counselors, the same reaction is likely to occur in those who are the listeners of emotional concerns such as dispatchers.

"It is believed that counselors working with trauma survivors experience vicarious trauma because of the work they do. Vicarious trauma is the emotional residue of exposure that counselors have from working with people as they are hearing their trauma stories and become witnesses to the pain, fear, and terror that trauma survivors have endured.

". . . This tension and preoccupation might be experienced by counselors in several ways. They might:

- avoid talking or thinking about what the trauma effected client(s) have been talking about, almost being numb to it

- be in a persistent arousal state

Counselors should be aware of the signs and symptoms of vicarious trauma and the potential emotional effects of working with trauma survivors." ("fact-sheet-9---vicarious-trauma.pdf," n.d.)

Following our experience on 9-11-01, it has become imminently clear that those who handle emergency 9-1-1 calls can experience the same sort of symptom pattern as those who experience trauma through direct exposure such as first responders or through military related trauma in our veterans. Clearly, the triggering events will be different but the physical and emotional reactivity will be the same.

Indeed, fourteen years after the 9-11-01 event, changes were made in the fifth edition of the Diagnostic and Statistical Manual of Mental Disorders (DSM-5). Among these alterations were changes to Criterion A for posttraumatic stress disorder (PTSD), related to the criterion that define specific events that qualify as traumatic.

The fundamental question explored was how to define a trauma by clarifying the emotional impact forth-coming from direct as compared to indirect trauma exposure. The authors note that: "Direct exposure includes experiencing a trauma firsthand or witnessing a trauma as it occurs to others. In contrast, indirect exposure may occur by learning about the violent or accidental death of a close associate, through secondary narrative accounts (e.g., in service-related professions), or through work-related media reports.

". . . Our review indicates that indirect exposure can lead to PTSD, although the probability of developing the disorder from indirect exposure is lower than that from direct exposure. Proximity to a trauma also increases risk, but this may be limited to direct exposure." (May & Wisco, 2016)

The following material is provided by a 9-1-1 dispatcher discussing the potential types of calls that are received across the context of a busy day at work or within the framework of the entirety of a career as a telecommunicator.

****

"As call takers we hear beatings, shootings, gasping, screaming, swearing, crying, rounds being fired, silence and then tears and sobbing. Callers, home alone, reach out to us with chest pains. We hear people take their last breath. We hear the agony in the voices of loved ones who find their deceased family members and we do our very best to calm the callers assuring them that help is on the way.

"Without real and visual information from the crime scene, car crash, house fire, SIDs death, homicide, and suicides, we are literally left to our own imaginations in an attempt to figure out what happened. Unlike first responders, we are back in the 'render assistance mode' almost immediately, without a chance to emotionally recharge or recover from what we have experienced.

"Adrenaline is initially our friend; it gives us the jolt to find the wherewithal to pick up the telephone, and confidently respond '9-1-1, where is your emergency?'. . . An interesting aspect of 9-1-1 work, I truly believe we get hooked on adrenaline. We need adrenaline. Our bodies thrive on adrenaline. But once we are on highly deserved and needed vacations, we spend the first week of our vacations sick due to adrenaline withdrawal.

"The very instant that call taker has verified the location and the chief complaint . . . those very fingers are moving at nearly light speed notifying dispatchers across the communication center of the issues. Without an audible queue the cops, paramedics and firefighters are sent to help the patient or victim. However, that takes time, minutes as their emergency vehicles dart through traffic. 'Help Is on the Way, Stay on the Phone While I Give You Some Instructions...'" (Rusk, 2014)

****

A historical argument has been made that unless one personally witnesses or directly experiences a trauma, the development of PTSD is not possible. Many still hold onto this false belief even though the DSM-5 criteria have altered to accommodate to this reality. Is there any wonder, based on the information provided in the above vignette, that continual exposure to highly emotionally charged material will exact a toll on the functioning and quality of life of the dispatcher?

"As a dispatcher experiences continual and overwhelming volumes of emotionally charged calls, the body, mind and spirit respond in ways to protect and help the person cope. Cumulative stress can affect work performance, work attendance, personal relationships and social relationships, in addition to presenting a multitude of physical manifestations." ("Dispatcher trauma: The unique stress of the job (and how to overcome it)

This is not to say there are not moments of humor, comradery, and group cohesion in this line of work. Rather it is the unexpected, the adrenaline rush that can come at any moment, the after effect of a tragedy, or the joy such as in the birth of a child in an unexpected place that creates the constant emotional churning that the dispatcher goes home with. An example of a humorous call is provided in the next vignette.

****

"This 4-year old boy has the cutest emergency ever. Following a lesson from his mother on what to do if he ever needs help from the police, he picks up the phone one day and calls 911, looking for help with his math homework. The dispatcher – after he figures out what's going on – is happy to help, talking subtraction with the young man until his mother walks in on the call.

Hey kid, we feel you. We all need a little help sometimes." ("4-year old boy calls 911 for help with his math homework| 7th Street District | H. Peter Ku, D.D.S. PA," 2014)

****

Like other first responders the pace of engagement for the dispatcher/telecommunicator is variable. In a natural disaster, one would expect the pace to be fast and quite demanding. The same can be said for nighttime shifts where more severe events are likely to occur. In general, there is no predicting what is to occur on a given shift.

Some perceive of this job as being highly routinized and devoid of creativity. Apparently, this is because the perceived goal is that of quickly identifying the pertinent issue and then determining what type of assistance, where warranted, needs to be directed to the specified location. The following story supports the perspective that innovation and imagination still play an integral part when dealing with crisis or trauma circumstances.

****

"Amanda Berlin only worked as a 911 dispatcher for about eight months when one particular call changed everything and earned her the title of bona fide hero.

"In April 2016, Amanda was working her usual shift in Tuscola County, Michigan when she received a concerning call from a cell phone. She could clearly hear a man and woman arguing, and the woman screaming — but the call was abruptly dropped.

Whoever called was in desperate need of help, but hung up before 911 could trace the location.

"Amanda tried calling the number back several times, but no one picked up. She knew exactly what was going on — there was a domestic violence incident taking place, and the woman was unable to safely communicate with Amanda over the phone. Thinking on her feet, Amanda quickly remembered a new emergency program called Smart911 — just weeks old at the time — that allows dispatchers to send text messages to victims.

"Amanda sent a text message to the caller's phone, asking if she needed help. 30 seconds later, Amanda was surprised yet relieved to get a text back: "Yes, please send help," it said. The woman was able to secretly text with Amanda, who then dispatched authorities to the home and arrested her attacker." ("911 Operator Gets Chilling Call For Help," n.d.)

****

A 2017 article measured baseline psychological measures between telecommunicators and police officers. The authors noted that: "Emergency telecommunications personnel (ETCP) form the hub of police agencies and persistently deal with distressing situations on a daily basis, making them highly susceptible to psychological and physiological ailments. . .

Results showed that ETCP self-reported greater levels of psychological stress compared with police officers ($p < .05$) for the majority of measures; ETCP experience excessive levels of stress and greater prevalence of chronic disease." (Ramey, Perkhounkova, Hein, Chung, & Anderson, 2017)

****

"Todd. . . told me his plane was being hijacked . . . he asked me if I knew what they wanted--was it ransom money or what. . . I could hear the commotion in the background and after we continued to talk, I'm thinking to myself, this is for real. This is a real hijacking situation.

"At one point, he thought I had left the phone. . . He was calling out my name and . . . I told him I would be there for him. And I stayed 'til the end.

". . . he said, 'Let's roll,' . . . And I was still on the line and the plane took a dive and by then, it just went silent.

"... I just could not believe that that plane had crashed. . . he gave me personal information regarding him and his family. . . And at the time when the plane crashed, they had announced over the radio that United Airlines Flight 93 had just crashed in Shanksville, Pennsylvania, and a guy put his hand on my shoulder and said, 'Lisa, you can release the line now. That was his plane.' And I said, 'No way'" And I kept calling his name and calling his name, hoping that he--just praying that anyone would come and pick up the phone. . ." ("The Inspirational Story of Lisa Jefferson: the Operator Who Took a Phone Call from United Flight 93 on 911 - Beliefnet," 2006)

****

A 2016 study examined the residual effects of stress manifested as burnout or exhaustion among 9-1-1-telecommunicators. ". . . Six emergency call centers in a state located in the Pacific Northwest were recruited to take an online survey during the month of April 2013. The survey collected self-reported information pertaining to job effort and reward, over-commitment, technostress, perceived control and colleague and supervisory support.

". . . A total of 156 telecommunicators were surveyed. . . We observed females having greater odds at taking sick days compared to male telecommunicators . . . We also found significant relationship between . . . the level of work commitment and its effects at home as well as the measure of physiological and physical indications of stress and sickness absenteeism." (Martin, 2016)

A survey published in the Journal of Traumatic Stress identified dispatchers' perception of 'worst calls' received in the following order: "unexpected injury or death of a child (16.4 percent of respondents), followed by suicidal callers (12.9 percent), shootings involving officers (9.9 percent) and calls involving the unexpected death of an adult (9.9 percent).

"Survey results showed that dispatchers experience high levels of "peritraumatic distress," the strong emotions felt during a traumatic event. Participants reported experiencing fear, helplessness or horror in reaction to nearly one-third of the different types of potentially traumatic calls.

"'Being a 911 dispatcher is generally considered a stressful profession,' Pierce said. 'However, the results from our study indicate the events typically handled by these first responders are also traumatic, and there can be adverse mental health effects. This implies a strong need to enhance prevention and intervention efforts.'" ("911 Dispatchers Suffer

PTSD Symptoms From Indirect Exposure to Traumatic Events," 2012)

The authors of the following 2017 study measured levels of cortisol among telecommunicators during incoming emergency calls. They postulated that: "Phone operators often deal with many absolute emergencies during the same shift, which may produce substantial hypersecretion of cortisol.

"A succession of days with elevated levels of cortisol can lead to serious diseases such as metabolic disorders including type two diabetes, and also depression and psychiatric disorders [22]. The impact of night shifts can also contribute to stress and to the alteration of the nictemeral cycle of cortisol, which can also lead to an increased morbidity and mortality [16,22]. Thus, the possibility of long-term adverse effects raises the question of the management of stress at work.

". . . The phone operators included in this study were representative of the overall population of emergency medical dispatchers. There was a greater increase in cortisol levels in response to stress in the men than in the women, as reported elsewhere [56] Another report showed that experienced individuals had a lower increase in cortisol levels and faster recovery compared to those without experience [57]." (Bedini et al., 2017)

****

"A Durham emergency dispatcher has been fired for not following procedure during a 911 call earlier this month that delayed response to a fatal fire. Marvin Jacobs, 74, died in the Aug. 17 fire at 110 Shantercliff Place. In a 911 recording of the call the dispatcher, Theresa Hopkins, repeatedly asks an unidentified female caller for the address of the fire.

"James Soukup, director of the Durham Emergency Communications, said that an investigation into what happened showed that Hopkins failed to follow procedure by not keeping the caller on the phone and not asking follow-up questions when she was unsure of the address.

"That could have included inquiring about nearby intersections or a phone number that could have been traced. Soukop also said that all the emergency equipment at the 911 center was working properly when the call came in but that an issue with the caller's telephone provider, Vonage, caused the address not to display on the 911 system.

"That and Hopkins' failure to get the information caused a delay of 4 minutes and

32 seconds, . . Investigators said they believe the fire started inside a vehicle Jacobs had been working on that evening. . . Durham authorities said Jacobs was the only person in the house at the time of the fire. Although his cause of death hasn't been determined, they said it appeared to be consistent with someone who was overtaken by smoke." ("Durham 911 dispatcher fired :WRAL. com," 2009)

****

Much like their direct contact first responder colleagues, telecommunicators more often than not, bring stress forthcoming from their outside life to the job as well as bringing the stress incurred through their work into their family life. The following authors discuss this phenomenon within the context of police work. I believe that it is just as applicable to the emergency dispatcher /telecommunicator.

They note that: "It has been said many times that you have to, 'Leave your home life at home and your work life at work.' Problems go with people wherever they go, therefore, being in law enforcement and observing death, violence, sexual assaults, and missing children (just to name a few) over and over again can spill over into an officer's home life, as well as their home life incidents can spill over into their job life.

"Use of alcohol and/or drugs, the start of or increase of domestic violence, the isolation of the officer causing the family to feel separated from the person even when that person is in the room with them may increase. The officer may feel that his/her family would never understand how he/she is feeling because they do not see the things he/she sees on the job. The sleepless nights, the sexual dysfunction, domestic violence, and divorce are all contributions of stress. Several researchers have agreed that the law enforcement profession has one of the highest rates for divorce, domestic violence, and suicide then that of the public they serve." (Carlan & Nored 2008)

"Counseling should be mandatory whether the traumatic incident takes place on duty or off duty because what affects the officer on duty, could ultimately impact the family in some way. Not only does the family possibly have to deal with the officer's bad day, they might have their own personal kind of stress associated with having a police officer in the family. . . Not to mention each time their loved one is due home, the family sometimes wonders if he/she will be in a bad mood today because of what the loved one endured while at work." ("INTRODUCTION - 1645.pdf," n.d.)

****

"HOUSTON — A 911 operator is accused of intentionally hanging up on callers during emergencies simply because she was not in the mood to help, according to Houston police.

". . . Williams had been employed as a telecommunicator with the Houston Emergency Center since July 2014, and supervisors began to notice that her logs revealed an abnormally high amount of 'short calls,' with a duration of less than 20 seconds.

Supervisors investigated the recorded call logs, and found that thousands of calls had been disconnected by Williams between Oct. 2015 and March 2016.

". . . Williams raised suspicion on March 12, specifically, when she allegedly hung up on several callers – the first call was ended immediately after she picked it up.

During the second call, an operator — identified as Williams — is heard answering 'Houston 911, do you need medical, police or fire?' When the male caller responded, "This is a robbery," Williams is heard sighing before hanging up, according to court documents.

". . . Police say Williams admitted to disconnecting the calls because she 'did not want to talk to anyone at that time.'

Investigators said Williams' actions prevented and interfered with the callers' ability to request assistance during an emergency and charges were filed against her. Williams' bond was set at $1,000.("Texas 911 operator accused of hanging up on callers: 'Ain't nobody got time for this' | WGN-TV," 2016)

****

There appears to be a sparsity of research pertaining to dispatcher/telecommunicator suicide. A 2017 article examined the relationship between emergency response services (ERS) personnel and suicide in Canada. The authors searched through multiple databases including: *"PubMed", "Web of Science", "Medline", "Psyc Articles", "Psyc Info", "Science Direct", "CINAHL,"* plus additional hand searching, and 40 articles were identified to meet search criteria and provide relevant information on this topic.

"The articles revealed that research has primarily focused on the traumatic stress and critical incidents encountered by emergency responders, while little research has been conducted specifically on suicide within these professions . . .The limited research that does discuss ERS suicide is largely restricted to law enforcement and military personnel. . . A research agenda is recommended to further investigate suicide among ERS within Canada, and the impact these suicides have on colleagues, families and friends." (Koopmans, Wagner, Schmidt, & Harder, 2017)

****

". . . Mercer understood early in her training that helping others would come at a price. She wouldn't come out unscathed . . . This is why her medicine cabinet is full of brown bottles, of carton boxes and torn tablets of prescription drugs.

. . . The nightmares started soon after a call she received in early 2012. . . She could hear sobbing between the shouts but her questions remained without reply. . . This was a problem because I had already taken all my sick days and so I had to keep working and it only made me worse. . . Cop movies, I couldn't watch them. I still can't. It just makes me freak out. I'm completely powerless. . . You're taught a lot of stuff, but not how not to get caught up in it.

". . . The stomach pumping was effective. The activated charcoals removed most of the sedatives in her digestive system and the ureteral stent cleared what was left in her kidneys. B vitamins are giving a boost to her liver functions. Walking hurts a lot. Breathing too. All these drains and fluids. I'm on the other side, now, . . . I'm one of them." ("The 911 Operator Who Needed Her Own Lifeline," 2015)

Summary

Dispatchers/Telecommunicators professionals serve as the gatekeepers to the providers of emergency services. The rapidly developing technology utilized by dispatchers has undoubtedly altered operational efficiency by reducing response time, thereby increasing the number of calls that can be processed per shift. Apparently, what is missing in this matrix is the impact that the increased workload has on the capacity of the human being to interface with potentially traumatic circumstances.

We have always known that the telecommunicator deals with traumatic circumstances and it has been assumed that vicarious trauma might be associated with this exposure. However, when an employee submitted a claim for benefits associated with this exposure, the rule of thumb was that that the claim was denied because the exposure was 'indirect.'

Alteration in the Diagnostic and Statistical Manual of Mental Disorders (DSM-5) related to the criteria necessary for the diagnosis of PTSD occurred in 2015. It is yet to be seen how this impacts future disability claims. If submitted claims are now successful, might the 'system' be more amenable to scientifically-based interventions that can remediate the effects of vicarious trauma? This would certainly become a motivating factor bringing about a new era in how compassion fatigue could be addressed.

References

4-year old boy calls 911 for help with his math homework| 7th Street District | H. Peter Ku, D.D.S. PA. (2014, November 17). https://fortworthtexasdentist.com/4-year-old-boy-calls-911-help-math-homework/

911 Dispatcher Job Description | 911 Operator Job Description. http://www.911 dispatcher edu.org/job-description/ 911 Dispatcher Jobs | 911 Operator Jobs. http:// ww.911 dispatcher edu.org/careers/

911 Dispatchers Suffer PTSD Symptoms From Indirect Exposure to Traumatic Events. (2012, March 29). http://www.ehstoday. com/eme-rgency-manage ment/911-dispatchers-suffer-ptsd-symptoms-indirect-exposure-traumatic-events

911 Operator Gets Chilling Call For Help. https ://littlethings.com/operator-text-message/?

utm_source=diq&utm_medium=Facebook&utm_campaign=shocking

Bedini, S., Braun, F., Weibel, L., Aussedat, M., Pereira, B., & Dutheil, F. (2017). Stress and salivary cortisol in emergency medical dispatchers: A randomized shifts control trial. *PLoS ONE*, *12*(5). https://doi.org/10.1371/journal.pone.0177094

Dispatcher trauma: The unique stress of the job (and how to overcome it). https://www.policeone.com/health-fitness/articles/171323006-Dispatcher-trauma-The-unique-stress-of-the-job-and-how-to-overcome-it/

Durham 911 dispatcher fired :: WRAL.com. http://www.wral.com/news/local/story/5888762/fact-sheet-9---vicarious-trauma.pdf. . http://www.counseling.org/docs/trauma-disaster/fact-sheet-9---vicarious-trauma.pdf

INTRODUCTION - 1645.pdf. https://shsu-ir.tdl.org/shsuir/bitstream/handle/20.500.11875/2056/1645.pdf?sequence=1

Koopmans, E., Wagner, S. L., Schmidt, G., & Harder, H. (2017). Emergency Response Services Suicide: A Crisis in Canada? *Journal of Loss and Trauma*, *0*(0), 1–13. https://doi.org/10.1080/15325024.2017.1360589

Martin, S. C. (2016, July 14). *Examining the Relationship Between Secondary Traumatic Stress and Sickness Absenteeism within 9-1-1 Emergency Call Centers* (Thesis). https://

digital.lib.washington.edu:443/researchworks/handle/1773/36709

May, C. L., & Wisco, B. E. (2016). Defining trauma: How level of exposure and proximity affect risk for posttraumatic stress disorder. *Psychological Trauma: Theory, Research, Practice and Policy, 8*(2), 233–240. https://doi.org/10.1037/tra0000077

New York City - Critical Shortage Of EMS Work ers. http://www.vosizneias.com/17032/2008/06/15/new-york-city-critical-shortage-of-ems-workers/

Newly hired 911 dispatchers begin training - City of Minneapolis. http://www.minneapolismn.gov/news/employees/WCMS1P-104789

Police, Fire, and Ambulance Dispatchers : Occupational Outlook Handbook: : U.S. Bureau of Labor Statistics. https://www.bls.gov/ooh/office-and-administrative-support/police-fire-and-ambulance-dispatchers.htm

Ramey, S. L., Perkhounkova, Y., Hein, M., Chung, S. J., & Anderson, A. A. (2017). Evaluation of Stress Experienced by Emergency Telecommunications Personnel Employed in a Large Metropolitan Police Department. *Workplace Health & Safety, 65*(7), 287–294. https://doi.org/10.1177/2165079916667736

Rusk, L. (2014, June 23). The Health Risks and Im pacts of Helping People On Their Worst Day. http://badgeoflifecanada.org/2014/06/23/the-health-risks-and-impacts-of-helping-people-on-their-worst-day-2/

Texas 911 operator accused of hanging up on callers: 'Ain't nobody got time for this' | WGN-TV. http://wgntv.com/2016/10/12/911-operator-accused-of-hanging-up-on-callers-aint-nobody-got-time-for-this/

The 911 Operator Who Needed Her Own Lifeline. (2015, September 10). http://narrative.ly/the-911-operator-who-needed-her-own-lifeline/

The Inspirational Story of Lisa Jefferson: the Operator Who Took a Phone Call from United Flight 93 on 911 - Beliefnet. http://www.beliefnet.com/inspiration/2006/06/i-promised-i-wouldnt-hang-up.aspx

Timm, A., & Ph.D, J. S. (2015). *Dispatcher Stress: 50 Lessons on Beating the Burnout*. Joe Serio Enterprises.

Chapter Eight

Correction Officers

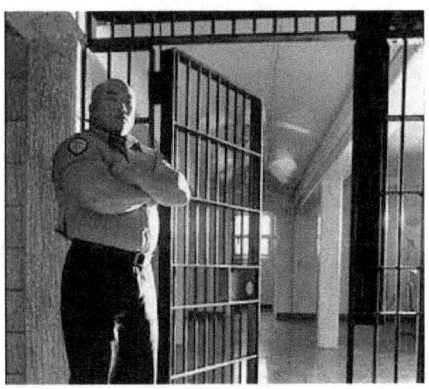

Lord, when it's time to go inside, that place of steel and stone, I pray that you will keep me safe, so I won't walk alone.

Help me to do my duty and please watch me on my rounds amongst those perilous places and slamming steel door sounds.

God, keep my fellow officers well and free from harm. Please let them know I'll be there too whenever there's alarm.

Above all, when I walk my beat, no matter where I roam, let me go back to whence I came, to family and home.

"In 2012, there were estimated to be around 469,500 correctional officers in the United States according to the U.S. Bureau of Labor Statistics. Most of these personnel are employed by federal, state or local governments working in our country's prisons and jails guarding the estimated 1.6 incarcerated adults in the United States.

Furthermore, according to the U.S. Bureau of Justice Statistics (BJS), 2,220,300 adults were incarcerated in U.S. federal and state prisons, and county jails in 2013 – about 0.91% of adults (1 in 110) in the U.S. resident population. The correctional officer oversees those individuals who have been arrested, awaiting trial, or have been sentenced to serve time. Typically, correctional officers are responsible for the following job duties:

1. **Enforce Rules and Keep Order:** Inside the prison or jail, correctional officers enforce rules and regulations. They maintain security by settling disputes between inmates, preventing disturbances, assaults, and escapes. Officers enforce regulations through effective communication and the use of progressive sanctions, which involve punishments, such as loss of privileges.

2. **Supervise Activities of Inmates:** Correctional officers supervise the daily activities of inmates, ensuring that inmates obey the rules. They must also ensure the whereabouts of all inmates at all times.

Officers also escort prisoners between the institution and courtrooms, medical facilities, and other destinations.

3. **Search for Contraband Items:** Officers search inmates and their living quarters for contraband, such as weapons and drugs. In addition, officers are responsible for screening visitors and incoming mail to ensure contraband is not brought into the prison or jail.

4. **Inspect Facilities to Ensure That They Meet Standards:** Correctional officers periodically inspect facilities. They check cells and other areas for unsanitary conditions, contraband, signs of a security breach (such as tampering with window bars and doors), and any other evidence of violations of the rules.

5. **Report on Inmate Conduct:** Correctional officers must report any inmate who violates the rules. If a crime is committed within their institution or an inmate escapes, they help law enforcement authorities investigate and search for the escapee. Correctional Officers are responsible for writing reports and filling out daily logs detailing inmate behavior and anything else of note that occurred during their shift.

6. **Aid in Rehabilitation and Counseling of Offenders:** As many prisons and jails are often incredibly understaffed, correctional officers with advanced training or college educations are often utilized in the rehabilitation and counseling of offenders. In addition, correctional officers also participate in the rehabilitation efforts by scheduling work assignments, counseling, and educational opportunities." ("Correctional Officer Duties & Responsibilites | Correctional Officer.org," updated 2017)

"Many facilities that utilize Correction Officers offer retirement benefits, although this may vary. At the federal level, officers typically work 8 hours per day, 5 days per week on rotating shifts. Due to jail and prison security being necessary around the clock, officers typically work all hours of the day and night, weekends and holidays. The average salaries of our Correctional Officers Salaries in the United States updated on July 23, 2017 is $32,309 per year." ("Correctional Officer Salaries in the United States | Indeed.com," updated 2017)

"In contrast, at the state level, Correction Officers tend to work a 12-hour shift which at times is extended to 16-hours when someone calls in sick. This change to 12-hour shifts is exemplified in a Florida 2011 announcement as follows: "Monticello – The Florida Department of Corrections will implement 12-hour shifts as a pilot program for its security staff at Jefferson Correctional Institution beginning June 10, 2011. Following a successful pilot, the Department will implement 12-hour shifts for correctional officers at its prisons statewide.

"Twelve-hour shifts will give correctional officers more time with their families and put more money in their wallets," said Florida Department of Corrections Secretary Edwin Buss. 'For taxpayers, it saves money because it reduces overtime and decreases the number of officers needed at the facility.'

"Twelve-hour shifts require correctional officers to work fewer days -- 182 days versus 260 days—and gives them every other weekend off. Officers will also be paid for an additional four hours of work each pay period. No correctional officers will lose their jobs, as savings will be achieved through attrition.

"Indiana, Alabama, Arkansas and Ohio are among the state prison systems that have implemented 12-hour shifts and have recommended them for other Corrections Departments. The program is expected to save nearly $170,000 annually at Jefferson CI alone. Jefferson Correctional was chosen as the pilot site because of its size, proximity to Tallahassee and strength of its warden and staff." ("Corrections Officers Going To 12 Hour Shifts - Prison Talk," 2011)

Unfortunately, the monetary saving and alleged benefits doesn't appear to correspond with the human wear and tear forthcoming from this level of sustained stress as well as its cumulative effects over prolonged periods of time. This is exemplified in the following vignette.

****

"(Claudia) Cass has just finished her overnight shift as a correctional officer at New Hampshire's State Prison for Men in Concord, where she spends upwards of 100 hours a week guarding medium- and maximum-security inmates. She has traded her blue polyester uniform for a dress, prepared to follow through on the "toughest decision" she has ever made: transferring legal custody of her 11-year-old son, Matthew, to her mother.

"I feel like a failure," says Cass, 42, a single mother. Her work in the prison had become so overwhelming that Matthew was often alone, cooking his own dinner and seeing himself off to school. 'I know I'm doing the right thing,' she says.

". . . for Cass and her fellow officers, the recurring nightmare is not a prison riot. It is falling asleep at the wheel after a series of 16-hour shifts. Or nodding off with your sidearm exposed while escorting a sick inmate to the hospital. Or even having to tell your child that you don't have time to be a mother.

". . . Concord Prison for Men needs 371 officers to operate normally. It takes 277 just to maintain critical operations. After years of budget cuts and attrition, the current staff at Concord is 203. And the inmate population has continued to grow.

"On at least a half-dozen occasions since May, Cass said, staff was so short she did the rounds on a 300-inmate floor by herself for the entire night. It's the largest single housing unit in the state and includes the prison's 96-member sex offender block. - The inmates know I'm working alone, Cass said." ("16-Hour Shifts, 300 Inmates to Watch, and 1 Lonely Son," 2014)

****

"Educational Requirements for a state Correctional Officer require a high school diploma or its equivalent. Post-secondary education is also a consideration for advancement purposes particularly by obtaining a college degree in criminal justice or sociology. Those who choose to become criminal justice majors take courses in crime and delinquency, criminal law and public management.

"To be employed within the Federal system, Correctional Officers must have either a 4-year college degree, three years of experience in a relevant field or some combination of education and experience. State and local employers typically do not require additional education if the officer has prior relevant work experience. In Florida, FDLE certification is required for both Law Enforcement and Department of Corrections. Some Officers are duel certified as both LO and CO.

"Once they are hired, federal and state correctional officers receive formal training at government training academies. Federal officers must complete 120 hours of special training in the first 60 days of work and then 200 hours of formal training within their first year of work. Some local correctional agencies also provide formal training but may utilize state facilities to do so. Additionally, the CO, depending on state regulations, may be further required to maintain current certification through 40 to 60 hours of yearly training.

Following the formal training period, correctional agencies then provide new hires with additional training on the job. While the type of on-the-job training varies between agencies, subjects that are taught may include relevant laws, firearms usage and self-defense tactics.

"Many employers administer a written exam, a background check and a drug test for job candidates prior to making a hiring decision. Employers may require candidates to meet minimum age requirements, usually between 18 and 21 years old. Federal agencies require officers to be appointed before they turn 37. New hires must also be U.S. citizens or possess a green card and have no felony convictions.

"According to the U.S. Bureau of Labor Statistics (BLS), correctional officers and jailers could expect to see a 4% job growth from 2014-2024, which was slower than average. Shorter prison terms and decreases in crime may be reasons behind this below-average job growth. Correctional officers and jailers made an average salary of $45,320 per year in May 2015." ("Correctional Officer," 2011)

As described in the following article, the pace of the Correction Officer's job is variable and filled with stressful uncertainties. The author notes that: "A corrections officer's day is anything but typical. One day at work may be quiet and uneventful while the next day could be filled with danger and violence. Corrections officers can be attacked or taken hostage at any moment, so officers must constantly be aware of their surroundings. If an inmate overpowers an officer and takes his weapon, the result can be catastrophic.

"At the beginning of the corrections officer's shift, there is usually a staff meeting to discuss various topics–the meeting is known as a "read off," and during the read off, officers are informed of their posts and duties for that day. While most posts are in the inmates' housing units, some posts involve admitting new inmates and getting their information processed and entered into the prison system.

"This 'intake' process is fast paced and requires a great deal of skill and experience in corrections. Inmates often arrive in an aggressive mood and will be less than cooperative during the intake process. Corrections officers hope that by treating the inmate with respect, they will be treated in a similar fashion. Sadly, however, that is rarely the case." ("Corrections Officer Jobs–What to Expect," updated 2017)

In order to provide you with material from Correction Officer's themselves, I have selected a range of officer reviews of the Illinois Department of Corrections. They report that: "A typical day at work was pretty much uneventful and grueling. I learned the value of working as a team and communicating to get things done as opposed to trying to shoulder too much of a burden individually. Management was diligent and never far away. My co-workers were cooperative and had good habits that influenced how I adjusted to the job. The hardest part of the job was staying motivated to do tiring work that had no real excitement. The most enjoyable part of the job was the feeling of accomplishment each day after work and understanding that I was earning my pay."

"Everyday I maintained safety and security throughout the institution. Each cell house was different but I never had any issues with the inmates. I felt the day went as smooth as you make it but there were alot of days I worked 16 hours so that became very tiresome. Although the money was great it was very time consuming and exhausting. All in all the job was great but I decided to relocate to California because I knew id be happier there. ." ("Working at Illinois Department Of Corrections: 60 Reviews | Indeed.com," updated 2017)

Let's take a look at the incarcerated population that Correction Officers are assigned to maintain rules and order with. As noted in the following display, the total number of those in the prison system, prison parole or probation hovers around 7 million.

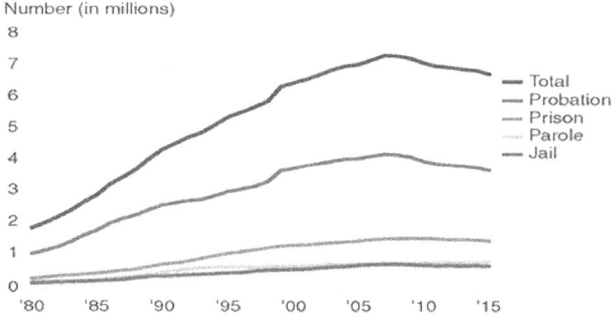

Total adult correctional population, 1980–2015

("Bureau of Justice Statistics (BJS) - Key Statistic: Total correctional population," updated 2017)

Understanding the nature of the incarcerated population is crucial in appreciating the environment that the correction officer must function in. A routinized daily pattern may suddenly erupt into a chaotic, out of control situation that may result in harm to those who are imprisoned as well as those who are charged with guarding and protecting them.

Because of this ever-present explosive potential, stress is a given factor in the lives of all involved in this environment including both prisoners and guards alike. Unfortunately, cumulative stress wreaks havoc on those who must endure it over extended periods of time. The severe consequences of this burden on the Correction Officer will be detailed in a later portion of this chapter.

As part of my effort to provide personal experience of those who work within this occupation, I elicited observations and comments from a former Correctional Officer (Kevin B). From time to time, I will insert his comments to further elucidate his perspective related to working in this profession.

I will also provide my own perspective related to cumulative stress matters. This consists of a number of variables contributing to the potential emotional lability of this often-diverse, incarcerated group of individuals. Among these factors are specific groups in our broader incarcerated population who are at increased risk for engagement in criminal offences including the following: chronic mentally ill; victims of early childhood and developmental trauma; homeless persons; drug and alcohol addicted individuals; members of minority groups.

My plan is to review each of these categories of incarcerated persons in some detail prior to exploring the emotional and physical impact that occurs among correctional officers. A 2017 piece provides an excellent synopsis of the chronic mentally ill issue in an article entitled: *Inside the nation's largest mental health institution: a prevalence study in a state prison system.* The researchers note that: "The mentally ill are overrepresented in correctional settings at estimated rates ranging from two to four times the general population.

"As a result, there are now ten times more individuals with Serious Mental Illnesses (SMI) in prisons and jails than there are in state mental hospitals. Incarceration of people with mental illness is a major public health issue, with social, clinical and economic implications. The balance between public safety and human rights has left corrections services with challenges in providing appropriate care for these patients." (Al-Rousan, Rubenstein, Sieleni, Deol, & Wallace, 2017)

As a mental health professional, I would like to reference the deinstitutionalization of mentally ill patients in this country beginning around 1955. One of the consequences of this action was the emergence of homelessness among this often-neglected population, which led to their increased involvement with the criminal justice system.

The results of a 2016 survey clearly convey the absolute crises that currently exists in this country pertaining to this vulnerable population. The author of the article noted that: "The number of last-resort psychiatric hospital beds that remain in state hospitals for patients whose treatment is not being, or cannot be, adequately addressed in a community setting has fallen to fewer than 12 beds per 100,000 population in the United States, the lowest level on record.

"This shortage has set off a domino effect of unmet demand that is reflected in such consequences as individuals in psychiatric crisis being boarded for days and even weeks in hospital emergency departments while they wait for hospital admission. It has also resulted in inmates in psychiatric crisis being wait-listed for weeks and months in jails and prisons as they wait for admission to forensic beds.

". . . In the first half of 2016, 37,679 staffed psychiatric beds remained in state hospitals, where individuals who are considered unsuccessfully treated and or too dangerous for other health care settings receive inpatient care. At 11.7 beds per 100,000 population, this represented a 17% drop from 2010 bed numbers and left fewer state hospital beds per capita in the United States than at any time since before the nation stopped treating mental illness as a crime in the 1850s.

Fast Facts

- Nearly 50% of the few state hospital beds remaining in service by 2016 (about 5.5 of the 11.7 per 100,000 people) were occupied by forensic patients charged with or

convicted of crimes, a population that has been exploding in many states.
- Despite a shift in state hospital budgets from civil to forensic treatment, most states maintain wait lists for their forensic beds, and some lists are months long.
- A growing number of states are resorting to hospital beds in corrections facilities ("beds behind bars") for criminal offenders because the number of available beds in the state mental health systems is inadequate to meet demand." (Carroll 2016)

****

"For most of his imprisonment, according to Nick, he received little treatment for his mental health and limited access to medicine that helped him. Long stretches in segregation made his illness worse. In an account confirmed by his medical records, he says his condition spiraled downward near the end of his sentence, when he attempted suicide and mutilated himself, biting a piece of flesh the size of a quarter from his own wrist. His desperate acts finally led to better care, including medicines that eased his symptoms, he says.

". . . Last year, 90 percent of the estimated 6,000 inmates with mental illness who were released from jails and prisons got little or no help from DMH as they tried to find treatment in the community, according to numbers provided by the state. Inmates like Nick Lynch don't even apply for DMH help; their conditions aren't considered serious enough under state criteria." ("Spotlight: Mental health and prisons, the new asylums" 2016)

****

Our next focal group is comprised of those who have experienced trauma early in their life and may have faced it as well throughout their developmental years. Unfortunately, our society is inclined to ignore events that occur in early childhood and thereafter unless they reach a level that is so glaring that it simply can't be ignored. In this sense, as a nation, we are motivated to intervene at a juncture that is far disconnected from the point that damage to the developing personality has taken place. We pay a tremendous price for this denial of the effects of early trauma as noted in the following 2017 study.

"This inquiry examined the developmental relationships between childhood traumatic experiences and drug use across the life-course. This was a national study which aimed to estimate the prevalence of nine types of childhood traumas including the cumulative number incurred and the associations between individual and cumulative number of traumas with drug use during adolescence, emerging adulthood, and adulthood.

The authors found that: "Nine typologies of childhood traumas: neglect; emotional, physical, and sexual abuse; parental incarceration and binge drinking; and witnessing, being threatened with, and experiencing violence . . . Each individual trauma was independently associated with either marijuana or cocaine use in adolescence, emerging adulthood, and/or adulthood. Childhood trauma is prevalent in the US and individual types as well as the total number experienced are significantly associated with Marijuana and cocaine use throughout the life-course." (Scheidell et al., 2017)

"Furthermore, the number of children exposed to traumatic incidents including violence in the United States is staggering. "According to the National Survey of Children's Exposure to Violence (NatSCEV), funded by the U.S. Department of Justice and the Centers for Disease Control and Prevention (CDC) and carried out by the University of New Hampshire's Crimes against Children Research Center, more than 60 percent of children surveyed had been exposed to direct or indirect violence during the 12 months prior to the survey.

"Nearly half — 46.3 percent — had been assaulted at least once in the past year, meaning they had experienced one or more of the following: any physical assault, assault with a weapon, assault with injury, attempted assault, attempted or completed kidnapping, assault by a brother or sister, assault by another child or adolescent, nonsexual genital assault, dating violence, bias attacks or threats.

"One in 10 had experienced some form of maltreatment, which includes nonsexual physical abuse, psychological or emotional abuse, child neglect and custodial interference. Other CDC research indicates that 1 in 4 girls and 1 in 6 boys are victims of sexual abuse. However, many experts emphasize that due to the stigma involved, sexual abuse is underreported." ("The toll of childhood trauma". 2014)

A point can be made here, based on the aforementioned information, that a common recourse to address the physical and emotional pain forthcoming from abuse is to seek to self-medicate the residual effects away. The driving force of choice to accomplish this objective is to utilize that agent which is most readily available.

"The physician, chief of Kaiser Permanente's revolutionary Department of Preventive Medicine in San Diego, CA, couldn't figure out why, each year for the last five years, more than half of the people in his obesity clinic dropped out. . . The mystery turned into a 25-year quest involving researchers from the Centers for Disease Control and Prevention and more than 17,000 members of Kaiser Permanente's San Diego care program.

". . . 'I misspoke,' he recalls, . . . Instead of asking, 'How old were you when you were first sexually active,' I asked, 'How much did you weigh when you were first sexually active?' The patient, a woman, answered, 'Forty pounds.' . . . 'It was when I was four years old, with my father.' . . . Of the 286 people whom Felitti and his colleagues interviewed, most had been sexually abused as children.

"As startling as this was, it turned out to be less significant than another piece of the puzzle that dropped into place during an interview with a woman who had been raped when she was 23 years old. In the year after the attack, she told Felitti that she'd gained 105 pounds. As she was thanking me for asking the question,' says Felitti, 'she looks down at the carpet, and mutters, 'Overweight is overlooked, and that's the way I need to be . . . The obese people that Felitti was interviewing . . . didn't see their weight as a problem. To them, eating was a fix, a solution." (Stevens, 2012)

Adverse Childhood Experiences were first identified in an extensive research initiative by the Centers for Disease Control and Prevention (CDC) and Kaiser Permanente in 1995. They studied the connections between childhood maltreatment and family dysfunction and adult health and mental health outcomes among over 17,000 people. This original ACE study drew several conclusions:

- when children are exposed to these 'adverse childhood experiences', the stress of this exposure may affect or disrupt the chemical and physical development of the child's brain and nervous system.
- when development of a child's brain and nervous system is disrupted, this affects the child's ability to cope with difficult or negative emotions and the child's cognitive and emotional development may be impaired.
- over time, the child will develop other coping mechanisms for dealing with negative or difficult emotions – this often plays out during adolescence, when the child may abuse drugs or alcohol as a coping

mechanism for the trauma experienced during childhood." ("ACES Paper for AFC CLE.pdf," 2014)

It is evident, even at this point in our exploration of vulnerable populations, that increased levels of incarceration are strongly associated with the experience of trauma occurring early and then cumulatively in life. I see this as a further extension of the effects that trauma has on our combat experienced veterans who develop PTSD symptomology.

Certainly, our corrections officers must function within a highly charged emotionally labile environment on a day to day basis throughout their careers. Similar principles would apply to our non-incarcerated citizens who have been exposed to varied form of trauma exposure.

****

"The daughter of an alcoholic, abusive father, Tamra Oman remembers trying to protect her mother from his violent outbursts, even though she was not yet in kindergarten. 'I remember him choking her over the sink. Spitting out blood. Blood coming out all over the place and landing on me,' Oman said, recounting one incident in her early childhood in Crown Point, Indiana. 'I remember going into this situation trying to save her. Trying to jump on top of him and save her. I can remember what I was wearing,' she continued. 'That's what trauma does. It also gets you stuck in those places.'

"For her part, Oman said the trauma she suffered as a young child set her on a path of self-destruction. She sabotaged success by dropping out of a series of colleges. She committed crimes.

"Oman finally ended up in prison, including two and a half years at Taycheedah and Burke women's prisons for forgery and writing bad checks. 'If you would've addressed my victimization as a child, I probably never would have ended up in prison,' Oman said. 'I became a perpetrator — not intentionally, but because that (trauma) never healed.'" ("Focus on traumatic childhood helps victims," 2016)

****

The next group subject to incarceration is found among those who find themselves subordinate to the 'war on drugs.' "Drug arrests now account for a quarter of the people locked up in America, but drug use rates have remained steady. Over the last 40 years, we have spent trillions of dollars on the failed and ineffective War on Drugs. Drug use has not declined, while millions of people—disproportionately poor people and people of color—have been caged and then branded with criminal records that pose barriers to employment, housing, and stability. ("The War on Drugs," 2017)

"As reported in the Boston Globe, 'The shortage of treatment resources in the community perpetuates a revolving door of release, relapse, and recidivism. Although there may be good substance-abuse treatment programs inside prisons and jails, there is a serious lack of support once inmates return to the community. An institutionalized population steps into a maze of underfunded and fragmented services.

"The numbers within the jail population alone are astounding. Nine million people are released from jail each year in the United States. Seventy-five percent have a history of substance abuse. After their release, 95 percent return to drugs and alcohol. Sixty-eight percent are reincarcerated within three years. This is a vulnerable and often neglected group with complex needs and considerations.

Many face poverty, homelessness, and mental health challenges.

"Even the briefest incarceration separates an individual from their daily lives and resources, often resulting in lost jobs, housing, transportation, and daily supports. Turning back to crime is frequently the most viable option to survive. And relapsing to drugs and alcohol may seem like the only way to find relief from the stress and loss." (30 & 2016,)

****

"I was a junkie before I ever landed on a prison yard, so it was only natural that I'd be indoctrinated into the heroin culture once I was confined within the walls of a federal prison. Drugs are incredibly ubiquitous in prison—marijuana, alcohol, and heroin seem to be the drugs of choice amongst the prisoners—surely because of their escapism properties. But you can't get high on your own supply.

"Anyone that has ever served a significant amount of time knows that getting out of your head is an indispensable part of keeping your sanity. But if you're selling you have to be careful and have some willpower or you'll use up all the drugs you're supposed to sell getting high with your celly. This could be the downfall of your whole operation. — *Biggie, an Aryan Nations member who served time in federal prison for cocaine conspiracy.* ("Prisoners on the Eight Rules of Dealing Drugs Behind Bars," 2016)

****

The numerous ways to do damage to the vulnerable tissue inside of the skull are quite numerous including: IED's; vehicle accidents; sports related head impact; etc. It is estimated that civilians alone will incur 1.7 million impacts per year that disturbs brain functioning. Another disturbing figure relates to an estimate that about 60 percent of incarcerated adults experienced at least one TBI prior to incarceration.

As noted in the following article: "These injuries, which can alter behavior, emotion and impulse control, can keep prisoners behind bars longer and increases the odds they will end up there again. Although the majority of people who suffer a TBI will not end up in the criminal justice system, each one who does costs states an average of $29,000 a year. With more than two million people in the U.S. currently locked up—and millions more lingering in the justice system on probation or supervision—the widespread issue of TBI in prison populations is starting to gain wider attention." (Harmon & Harmon,)

A 2017 study found that individuals with a history of traumatic brain injury are more likely to be incarcerated that those who have not incurred such an impact. The authors report that: "Individuals with TBI may exhibit more aggression and impulsivity and researchers have questioned whether these behavioral changes make it more likely that individuals with TBI will become involved with the criminal justice system. . . The researchers also found that men who had multiple TBIs had an even higher risk of incarceration than men with only one TBI. . . This may be just the tip of the iceberg as our study focused only on people with more serious TBI." (Peters, 2017)

****

"On Feb. 11, 2005, (Kenny) Eastridge's Humvee drove over a double-stacked anti-tank mine. Eastridge says he was blown from his position in the gun turret and landed unconscious some distance from the vehicle. . . The next day, back on base, his friends in Third Platoon noticed a clear liquid leaking from his ears. The company medic told him it was 'probably cerebral fluid.' . . . I was never taken back to the hospital. ... They just brought me back and when my leg healed, they put me back out on missions. . . I'm still having headaches and memory problems."

"Eastridge's medical records from his first tour in Iraq have been lost and there is no way of checking his version of his treatment, or lack of it, against the army's own records -- although other members of Third Platoon have confirmed his account of the IED and of the clear fluid leaking from his ears.

"The loss of the medical records meant that once Eastridge came home, there was no record of him having suffered a TBI in Iraq. . . Eastridge went on to serve another combat tour, and was exposed to several bomb blasts. He is now serving 10 years in prison for his role in a string of crimes in Colorado Springs in 2008, including the violent assault of a teenage girl and the murder of a fellow soldier." ("Brain Wars," 2010)

****

The next distinct and significant group contributing to the incarcerated population consists of those who were formerly homeless. The relationship between homelessness, mental illness, and criminal justice has been well correlated in the past. ("03Occupational Stressors.pdf," 2008) The investigators found that: "Inmates who had been homeless (that is, those who reported an episode of homelessness anytime in the year before incarceration) made up 15.3% of the U.S. jail population, or 7.5 to 11.3 times the standardized estimate of 1.36% to 2.03% in the general U.S. adult population."

"The results further suggest that the correlation between homelessness and mental health difficulties are almost entirely facilitated by alcohol use, drug use, and prior violent victimization. Missing in the discussion is the critical word trauma, which in my mind is the underlying causative factor leading to homelessness in the first place." (Fox, Mulvey, Katz, & Shafer, 2016)

****

"(Peter) Starks describes the experience of a typical inmate leaving jail or prison and confronting a mound of paperwork. Fill this out and go here for treatment. Fill that out and go there for housing. 'Before you get there you've got skid row, where all your healing needs are met,' Starks says. 'The dope man is going to get paid. So getting to you people — it's not going to happen.'

"Starks may have had little use for an apartment, living instead for eight years on the stage at MacArthur Park and 13 on the sidewalk in front of a drop-in center. But ultimately, he was housed — by Amistad de Los Angeles . . . There, he said, he learned to deal not just with drugs and illness, but with underlying issues that exacerbated those problems, like resentment, anger and trauma stemming from his time in combat in Vietnam.

"For him, homelessness was merely one symptom of the central challenge, which is reentry: a return to society after a long period of incarceration, with the other symptoms, like substance abuse and emotional trauma, still intact." (Greene, 2016)

****

Another highly significant aspect of our prison population consists of those inmates who meet criteria for the diagnosis of PTSD. A 2016 study found evidence for the presence of PTSD in 48% of the prison sample as compared to 4% of the general population sample. In breaking this down further, the investigators found that 70% of imprisoned women experienced childhood sexual abuse with a parallel rate of 50% for men.

The findings revealed that: "In the general population sample, participants who had only 1 type of trauma exposure had a 0% likelihood of current PTSD, whereas those with 6 or more other trauma types had a 12% likelihood. In the prison sample, those with only 1 type of trauma exposure had a 17% percent likelihood of current PTSD, whereas those exposed to 6 or more other trauma types had a 64% chance of PTSD."

The researchers concluded that: "Cumulative trauma predicts current PTSD in both general population and prison samples, even after controlling for sexual trauma. PTSD appears to develop generally as a function of exposure to multiple types of interpersonal trauma, as opposed to a single traumatic event." (Briere, Agee, & Dietrich, 2016)

The previous study mentioned the disproportionate degree of PTSD found among incarcerated women.

Another 2016 study found that: "The theoretical portion of this primarily feminist research identified and developed what has become known as *pathways theory*, documenting the excessively high risk of experiencing adverse life events, particularly abuse victimization, among offending women and girls (compared with nonoffending women and girls and compared with offending men and boys).

"In brief, pathways theory, explored mostly with women and girl offenders, posits that adverse life events, particularly traumatic events such as child sexual abuse and intimate partner abuse, are risk factors for offending." (Lurigio, Belknap, Lynch, & DeHart, 2016)

In regard to minority representation in prisons, "According to the US Census Bureau, 3.3% of Iowa's population is African-American, in contrast to 26% in the state prison system. Mental health challenges, substance use disorders, and HIV/AIDS disproportionately affect African-Americans in correctional settings, consistent with our findings. Minority inmates had mental illness rates generally similar to Whites, but Whites were more likely to have more than one mental illness diagnosis.

"Of interest, female Hispanic inmates were more likely to have three or more mental conditions in contrast to their White and Black counterparts. Women inmates, especially younger ones, were more likely than men to be diagnosed with a larger variety of mental disorders in this analysis. Women in general were at greater risk than men to be diagnosed with mental illness during incarceration." (Al-Rousan et al., 2017)

Additionally, factors related to sexual minorities among US inmates was explored from data obtained from the National Inmate Survey, 2011-2012. The authors concluded that: "Sexual minorities (those who self-identify as lesbian, gay, or bisexual or report a same-sex sexual experience before arrival at the facility) were disproportionately incarcerated: 9.3% of men in prison, 6.2% of men in jail, 42.1% of women in prison, and 35.7% of women in jail were sexual minorities.

"The incarceration rate of self-identified lesbian, gay, or bisexual persons was 1882 per 100 000, more than 3 times that of the US adult population. Compared with straight inmates, sexual minorities were more likely to have been sexually victimized as children, to have been sexually victimized while incarcerated, to have experienced solitary confinement and other sanctions, and to report current psychological distress." (Meyer et al., 2017)

I've provided an incomplete review of the varied aspects of the institutionalized population. For example, I haven't discussed gang related contributions to the undercurrents that constantly swirls within the prison environment. Neither have I discussed in detail the disproportionate representation of Black and Hispanic members of the overall community. Independent of this, I do believe that I've made the point that working within the prison setting as a correction officer over time likely has emotional and physical impact on those who serve.

At this point, I'd like to shift focus back to the correction officer, focusing on the effects that cumulative stress has on his/her health and overall functioning. Additionally, I'll briefly focus on the economic impact that PTSD ultimately has on society.

I will follow with discussion pertaining to the ripple effects that this occupation has on: family function including the following: intimate partner violence; addictive issues; suicide. In order to stay within the confines of the chapter I made an effort to select the most salient and recent reference to illustrate what I wish to convey.

****

"Activity event log for each holding unit are maintained by the Correctional Officer on the assigned post. Every event no matter how small is recorded. I see this as a CYA operation. Kevin B

****

"We face some of the ugliest statistics of mortality as correctional officers. Perhaps you have seen these, they are fairly commonly cited online in other articles, but just in case you need a reality check here it is:

- "Correctional Officers (CO's) have the second highest mortality rate of any occupation.
- 33.5% of all assaults in prisons and jails are committed by inmates against staff.
- A CO's 58th birthday, on average, is their last.
- A CO will be seriously assaulted at least twice in a 20-year career.
- On average, a CO will live only 18 months after retirement.
- CO's have a 39% higher suicide rate than any other occupation,
- And have a higher divorce and substance abuse rates then the general population." ("Beating The Odds,")

Let's begin with an article that focuses broadly on the economic impact related to prevalence and societal costs associated with PTSD. Those personnel who are: "affected by burnout took more sick-leaves and this affected adversely their remuneration as they lost 3.1% of their annual wages. Their expenses spent on user fees for medical services were 3 times higher. Their monthly expenses spent on medications were 3.14 times higher than those of people without the burnout syndrome." (Stoyanova & Harizanova, 2016)

It is important to understand that within the correction officer's environment, the cumulative aspects of frequent exposure to trauma have a deteriorative effect over time. The following study sought to investigate: "the degree to which correctional officers experience emotion while on their shifts, and how those emotions may translate into stress, divorce, substance abuse issues, domestic violence, and high mortality rates upon retirement.

". . . The findings of this study show a high percentage of respondent's report feelings of anxiety throughout a shift at work. Further, the findings show that the participants consistently report a disconnect between felt and expressed emotions while at work." (Grammatico, 2017) Suffice it to say, these are the very ingredients simmering in the 'slow cooker' for burnout, compassion fatigue and ultimately PTSD.

". . . Death, accidents, criminal behavior, inhuman acts, threats to the individual and other engagement, while more measured in their accumulation, may result in severe personal adverse outcomes. The harm, while often of gradual accumulation, can terminate a career, bring irreparable harm, and cause the loss of skills and service the individual once provided." ("The Reality of PTSD in Police/Law Enforcement, Emergency Responders, and Custody Services - viewcontent.cgi," 2016)

****

Once you establish a CO to inmate form of respect or status, inmates will stop the manipulation games. Unfortunately, this is not the case for every CO as it seems that some officers always have a hard time with inmates because they try too hard to force respect. Still, you always have to be on guard.

"The inmate is thinking, what can I get away with or slip pass the CO? I learned to establish my pet peeves up front. Inmates respect that mentality, and some of the hard-core inmate's hint that vocal dialog to new officers. Let us know where you stand! Most of the time, (this statement will vary day to day) the most stress I had experienced came from fellow staff and upper management as well as being confined alone on a 12 to 16-hour shift." Kevin B.

****

Similar to other first responders, stigma and a creed of masculinity too often block afflicted officers from seeking assistance. The following researchers sought to elicit officers' perceptions of, and responses to, stressful and traumatic events. "Results indicate that many officers have experienced traumatic events, and/or know a fellow officer who has experienced trauma on the job. Yet, these officers are reluctant to disclose their experiences to their agency.

"Moreover, results indicate that many officers are hesitant to seek help within their agency, suggesting barriers such as pervasive stigma." (Fleischmann, Strode, Broussard, & Compton, 2016)

I'll now shift to the effects that this ongoing stress may have on the well-being and health status of the career employee. As noted in a recent 2017 article, the authors report that: "Correctional officers have one of the most stressful jobs in our society yet have been largely neglected in occupational safety and health research.

"Correctional officers are at increased risk for cardiovascular, musculoskeletal, and posttraumatic stress disorders, and suffer from suicide rates nearly triple of those observed among the general population and in other related occupations. Actuarial tables indicate a 12–15-year life expectancy gap between correctional officers and the general population." (Henning et al., 2017)

Among the prominent comorbid conditions to compassion fatigue and PTSD, sleep disturbance appears to be quite prevalent among correction officers likely due to varying shifts, ongoing stress and cumulative fatigue. The investigators found that: "28% and 45% of the sample reported suffering from Apnea and insomnia, respectively. The following authors note that: "Over half of the sample reporting sleeping less than 2 hours between shifts and being constantly fatigued. We found significant associations between exposure to critical incidents and sleep problems. Prison workers are in desperate need of help to improve their sleep." (James, Todak, & Best, 2017)

"Finally, the following authors found that correctional officers were at risk for nonfatal injury due to overexertion. Their job duties include a variety of activities that increase their risk for strained muscles, sprains and other musculoskeletal injuries due to the use of excessive physical effort, awkward body postures and/or static postures. Such activities include restraining inmates or breaking up fights, moving heavy furniture or equipment during contraband searches and standing for a prolonged time to supervise inmates." (Konda, Tiesman, Reichard, & Hartley, 2013)

****

"During the course of my 15-year career as a correctional officer at the jail I have watched countless videos of inmate fights, stabbings, killings. That's part of training. Once in a while they show us videos of staff getting assaulted, or we read on the Internet about such assaults all over the country. I have also witnessed many such incidents first-hand, probably about 10 serious ones (inmates were killed or had to receive medical care at a hospital), and another 30-40 garden-variety assaults and group fights.

"I myself have been seriously assaulted three times—cold-cocked while trying to restrain an inmate, kicked, and cut with a shank. I've also responded to three inmate suicides. I had to perform CPR on one of them, even though he was cold—too far gone. Really, nothing that I see at work upsets me anymore. The only thing that gets to me is staff who are too soft or weak.

"My wife tells me that I've become hard, uncaring. When I tell her that dead inmates don't bother me, she is shocked. The other day she asked me how I can possibly deal with murders and suicides and not blink an eye.

"She asked, "Does this come with the job or are you just heartless?" My children seem to be a little afraid of me as I am strict and fly off the handle easily. Once in a while I have a nightmare about the jail. It causes me to bolt straight up in bed sweating, my heart racing." ("Occupational Exposure to Primary and Secondary Trauma in Corrections," 2014)

****

As noted in the above vignette, the family is a primary recipient of the after-effects of stress brought home from the job. The dual pulls from the work setting and the role expectations from the family can add to the officer's perception of gradual loss of control. Additionally, family members are vulnerable to the effects of secondary trauma from exposure through the 'primary carrier.'

As found in a 2015 article: "When the tipping point of conflict between the two is reached, a negative impact on employee well-being can result. Within correctional environments, the psychosocial well-being of officers is critical given the potentially significant impact of having a 'bad day on the job.'

". . . Findings indicate strain and behavior-based work–family conflict and family–work conflict were significantly related to both job stress and job satisfaction. Family and supervisory support were uniquely related to job stress, whereas supervisory support, education, and ethnicity were uniquely related to job satisfaction." (Armstrong, Atkin-Plunk, & Wells, 2015)

> ***********************
>
> "We never saw each other except in passing. Twelve-hour shifts and mandatory overtime, additional required trainings and weapons qualifying, being called in on his day off, rotating and unpredictable schedules – he is truly married to his job as much as he is married to me. . . If new recruits were aware of how daunting the statistics for corrections officers are, they probably would never have applied.

"CO's have a 39 percent higher suicide rate than any other occupation. Their life expectancy is only 58 years: that's 20 years less than the average American. CO's have high rates of heart attacks and alcoholism. Add to that a higher-than-average divorce rate and a higher prevalence of mental illnesses such as PTSD, anxiety and depression, and you can clearly see how job stress directly affects your loved ones and your relationship.

". . . Despite these statistics the hardest part for me is knowing that my spouse, this person I love as much as my children and life itself, could be assaulted at work and sustain a life-threatening injury *from doing his job.*

"Every day he goes to work with the intention of protecting staff and inmates from harm. He takes pride as a public servant who keeps the worst of the worst behind bars to keep society and his family safe. As I watch him iron his uniform and walk out the door in his boots and epaulets, I hold my breath and pray that today won't be that day." ("What's it like being a CO spouse?," 2014)

****

In researching information pertaining to correction officer addictions, domestic violence and suicide, I notice a sparsity of formal research on these topics. I wonder why this is so when the dated material seems so impactful. As noted in the earlier vignette, suicide rates at 39%, life expectancy at 58 years, high rates of alcoholism and heart attacks would, I would think, send shudders throughout the land. Who on earth would want to sign up for a career with these odds so stacked against them?

It is an interesting comment that first responders are the first to arrive to a crisis and typically the last to request help for an addiction. "A recent study by the U.S. Department of Health found that 23% of first responders are addicted to drugs and alcohol versus 8% of the general population. . . These problems not only harm first responders, but also the people officers are supposed to protect. Substance abuse impairs judgement in emergency situations, endangers lives, and adds to the public's growing mistrust of police officers and other emergency workers.

"Instead of addressing addiction problems, public safety organizations sweep them under the rug and maintain traditional work cultures that discourage asking for help. Scared to show any sign of weakness, public safety officers often keep their problems secret." ("First Responders and Addiction," 2015)

Unfortunately, 'emotions' tend to be perceived as being equivalent to a dirty word in many correctional settings. "Officers are drilled on codes, procedures, and handling weapons. But they are not taught how to process the daily drudge and the intense and traumatic experiences they encounter.

"Coping mechanisms come in all shapes and sizes. Healthy and unhealthy ones become the everyday practice of LEOs. Alcohol is a depressant and will dull thoughts and feelings, while also causing some to feel even more invincible or simply block out all the emotions they cannot process.

". . . The flux of emotions, along with physiological effects, creates a perfect storm if that officer doesn't have a healthy way to decompress. Add to the equation a culture that encourages camaraderie over a few drinks and you can end up with an officer on the road to alcoholism." (Morel, 29, & Said, 2016)

****

"The job is toxic and if you don't take care of yourself, it will catch up to you," said John Marx, a former longtime Colorado law enforcement officer and founder of The Law Enforcement Survival Institute.

"Jode Sprague once fancied himself the typical macho cop. He didn't talk about his feelings. He didn't cry. "We don't want to appear weak, the Colorado homicide detective said in an interview. During his decades in policing, he'd lost close friends in shootings. He'd seen hundreds of bodies. In 2003, he killed a man who tried to stab his partner. The emotional toll led him to seek the comfort of booze.

"Several years ago, Sprague saw no hope. He decided to end it. He left a suicide note, took an overdose of sleeping pills and crawled into bed. His then-wife found the note and called for help. Paramedics revived him.

"It's just not normal. You can't keep those things inside,' said Sprague, who is back on the job and serves on his department's peer support team. 'The alcohol just deadens the pain, but as soon as you sober up, you still have the same problems.'" ("They drink when they're blue," 2012)

****

Let me first apologize for referencing a police vignette as an example of alcohol difficulties. Quite frankly, I couldn't find a similar citation in the correction officer literature. I'll now shift to an issue that's frequently associated with alcohol dependence, which is Intimate Partner Violence (IPV). Unfortunately, I must also include a police officer focus on the following topic as well. A 2013 article explores why law enforcement personnel have a tendency to ignore violence against women when the perpetrator is another officer.

"Mark Wynn, a former Nashville police lieutenant who advises departments worldwide on the model rules. 'Whenever you are aware of a crime and you don't hold someone accountable, then you are colluding with a criminal. Is that what we want in the ranks of law enforcement?'

"Experts believe domestic abuse to be the most commonly unreported crime. Police officers can be particularly dangerous because of their access to guns and special training in fighting and controlling those who challenge them. Yet their victims often do not report abuse because they fear retaliation and they believe that their abuser's colleagues, as well as prosecutors, will not take their complaints seriously.

"It's been covered up since the beginning of time," said Penny Harrington, a former police chief in Portland, Ore. Ms. Harrington said that even when accusations are reported, prosecutors may be reluctant to pursue them because they need officers to testify in other cases and do not wish to create ill will. ("Departments Slow to Police Their Own Abusers," 2013)

****

"Speaking from my personal experience, most Law Enforcement Officers, could not, would not, and should not work as an Correctional Officer. You are locked in behind the bars and remain confined until someone opens those locks. I have some law enforcement buddies that told me face to face, 'hell no, I will never work inside-inside. The most I will go, is booking. That's it.' I then laugh and say, you pussy, inmates are easy to deal with. At least, I can see what's coming.

"But truthfully, this is not so in all cases. If something goes down, there is nowhere to run. Then that inmate or inmates, have the attitude of payback like: 'I'm going to make your life even more hell.' This is coming from their confinement, lack of privileges, or because I am the damn CO.

"In turn, my attitude becomes one of: now, you are on my shit list. I going to make your buddies life hell too. I'll lock the biggest and meanest inmate up in confinement. Inmates then by the Miracles of God, seem to have a change of heart. I had to do just that, more than once. In one case, I locked two up. Never had a problem from the cell again. New inmates were quick to learn the rules. Don't mess with Officer B." Kevin B.

****

The following 2012 article presents statewide data pertaining to correctional officers' attitudes and personal experiences with domestic violence. "Online surveys were administered to Florida correctional officers asking a series of questions, including their beliefs and attitudes about the prevalence of domestic violence among colleagues, and their childhood and adult experiences with domestic violence.

"Results . . . revealed that 33 % of respondents knew about correctional officers who had committed unreported domestic violence; 30 % reported that they had directly experienced domestic violence as children; and over 11 % reported that they had been physically violent with an intimate partner. Multivariate statistics showed that age, race, and childhood experiences with domestic violence were significantly related to correctional officers reporting being physically abusive to an intimate partner or family member." (Valentine, Oehme, & Martin, 2012)

****

"A Nevada Department of Corrections guard has been arrested on suspicion of a domestic battery charge. Joseph Bartlett, 28, of Reno, was arrested Thursday morning at 12:05 a.m. after Carson City Sheriff's Office deputies conducted a warrant service at the Northern Nevada Corrections Center for felony domestic battery with strangulation.

"According to the Reno Police Department arrest report, Bartlett had allegedly gotten into a verbal fight with the victim near the 2500 block of Melody Drive in Reno around 11:30 p.m. The victim told witnesses during the fight Bartlett asked her for the dog leash and proceeded to place the leash around her neck and tighten it. The victim told police she couldn't breathe for about 20 to 30 seconds before he let go.

"Reno police officers and Carson City deputies made contact with the suspect at the Correction Center where he was arrested without incident. Bartlett was arrested on domestic battery with strangulation and bail was set at $15,000." ("Update," 2017)

****

The next topic is an uncomfortable one pertaining to the way in which a particular profession is viewed by others as well as by peers. In the world of law enforcement unfortunately, correction officers are inclined to be seen as being 'low in the barrel.' The following article compares firefighters to correction officers in regards to how they are perceived by society and peers.

"While firefighters successfully labor to sustain their reputation as 'America's heroes' . . . correctional officers must work to overcome their reputations as 'professional babysitter' and the scum of law enforcement. Emerson and Pollner (1976) extended the concept of dirty work to include aspects of the job that are shameful, disliked, or serve to challenge the self-image of the worker. . . Physical taint takes place in jobs associated with dirt, garbage, sewage, death, bodily fluids, or dangerous conditions.

"Correctional officer work is dirty on a number of levels. . . Officers chaperone inmates to the bathroom (to ensure inmates do not hide contraband on or in their bodies) and conduct inmate "strip outs" after visitation sessions. . . Officers also are responsible for cleaning up the (literal and figurative) messes occasioned by inmates who, for instance, swallow foreign objects, sexually abuse each other, trash their cells, throw food at officers, or play with their feces.

"One officer explained, 'I'm sick of people thinking we're all bad, killing people left and right.' Another said, 'They think that we're part of the punishment, that we're uneducated, big, mean people barking out orders. . . I've even had people ask me if we beat people! . . . Officers not only felt denigrated by the general public but also, in what appeared to be an even greater insult, felt disparaged by members of other law enforcement occupations. They said: "Police officers don't consider us to even be in their same category." ("MCQ287898.qxd - Sexuality-Masculinity-and-Taint-Management-Among-Firefighters-and-Correctional-Officers-Getting-Down-and-Dirty-With-Americas-Heroes-and-the-Scum-of-Law-Enforce-ment.pdf," 2016)

Suppressing the daily fear and accompanying emotions over time plays havoc with one's sense of well-being. The unofficial correction officer's motto, "Eight and the Gate" speaks loudly to the aspect of denial that comes into play in this particular occupation. Variable shifts, exposure to violence among a volatile prison population, loss of empathy for those they are assigned to guard, a macho culture that resists sharing with colleagues all lead to burnout, compassion fatigue and then PTSD.

A 2013 study focused on earlier research related to the elevated risk of suicide within law enforcement occupations. "The present study examined the proportionate mortality for suicide in law enforcement in comparison to the US working population during 1999, 2003-2004, and 2007, based on Centers for Disease Control and Prevention's National Institute for Occupational Safety and Health National Occupation-al Mortality Surveillance data. We . . . focused on two specific law enforcement occupational categories-detectives/ criminal investigators/ police and corrections officers.

"Suicides were also explored by race, gender and ethnicity. . . Detectives/criminal investigators/police had the higher suicide risk (an 82% increase) compared to corrections officers (a 41% increase). . .The results included significantly increased risk for suicide among detectives/criminal investigators/ police and corrections officers, which suggests that additional study could provide better data to inform us for preventive action." (Violanti, Robinson, & Shen, 2013)

I've searched for the origins of the 39% figure related to correction officers suicide rate as compared to the general public. I believe that I found it in a 1997 study that focused on this topic as noted in the following article:

"Research on factors such as stress, burnout, and work dissatisfaction has often found high levels of these problems among guards. The present study analyses data from 21 states to ascertain whether guards are at risk of suicide. The results of a multivariate logistic regression analysis indicate that the risk of suicide among guards in 39% higher than that of the rest of the working age population." (Stack & Tsoudis, 1997)

****

"Michael Van Patten's 18-year-old son came home to find his dad crouching on the kitchen floor, gun in hand, a nearly empty bottle of gin by his side, tears running down his cheeks. Trevor grabbed the weapon, ran up to his room, shut the door and didn't speak to his dad – or anyone – about the incident for 13 years.

"For Michael, this was the build-up of nearly three decades working as a corrections officer at the Oregon state penitentiary. "The only way I knew how to deal with it was to eat a bullet.

"Right now, we're about where the military was 10, 15 years ago when it comes to them dealing with PTSD," . . . Nearly 20 of his fellow officers have committed suicide since he started working in corrections. He nearly became a statistic himself.

"... In the years and months leading up to his attempted suicide, Michael suffered from all the typical symptoms of PTSD: insomnia, cold sweats, phantom violence while asleep. He worked out obsessively and self-medicated with alcohol. He didn't even know what PTSD was at the time. That's partly because it's not something that COs talked about. The culture is tough and macho, and any sign of vulnerability, especially a mental health diagnosis, carries stigma." ("'Prison guards can never be weak': the hidden PTSD crisis in America's jails | US news | The Guardian," 2015)

****

Summary

I began this chapter with a description of the correction officer's responsibilities related to a diverse group of incarcerated prisoners. Descriptions of some aspects of this, at times, volatile population was included in order to better understand the challenges the correction officer faces on a daily basis. It is no wonder that the CO would be hesitant to display any indicators of emotion before members of this volatile and at times, explosive group.

To show weakness, empathy, kindness or other qualities of human compassion could prove to be fatal in such a diversified prison environment. The prevailing attitude becomes one of 'protect and defend' both among those who are imprisoned, as well as those who guard and protect them.

Fear and its accompanying companion, anxiety, become prevalent. Over time, this wreaks havoc with the natural balance in the afflicted human. Unlike other mammals, human beings have lost the ability to automatically re-establish a critical homeostatic balance. Might this be the reason that the correction officer will likely live only 18 months after retirement? Might this be the reason that CO's have a 39% higher suicide rate than other occupations? Might this be the reason that the CO is at increased risk for cardiovascular, musculoskeletal, and other physical and mental disturbances?

Perhaps the change to twelve-hour shifts that sometimes turn into 16-hours is a contributing factor to the vulnerability of the CO to cumulative stress factors, including sleep disorders and other physical maladies. Alternatively, being alone in a dangerous environment for this sustained period of time might also affect the individual over time.

What might be done to alter this terrible dismal picture? As described in earlier chapters, we are advancing in our knowledge of how trauma effects the mind and body of humans. I've personally come to the perspective that trauma of various kinds is the root cause for a preponderance of mental illness.

Diagnosis is based on symptoms presented by the afflicted individual. If these symptoms are the results of unresolved trauma, we end up missing the primary factor in a futile effect to put out the brushfires caused by the primary issue. Suffice it to say, I pay little attention to diagnosis nowadays in my quest to end the nightmare of compassion fatigue/PTSD.

As you might already guess from reading earlier chapters, there is a solution, both for those who are imprisoned, as well as those who guard them. Specifically, I'd would like to implement RESET Therapy research within the context of a correction setting. Were this to demonstrate efficacy, broader implementation would be a next step.

Perhaps there is an alternative way to intervene with the offender population. By quieting and calming the emotional center of the brain through non-invasive means, we may come to alter consequent behavior. For the Correction Officer, I would speculate that clearing the accumulated stress following a shift or perhaps doing so on a weekly basis would reverse some of the startling statistics associated with their occupation. Similar to the hierarchy within police departments, administration can facilitate such a clearing of accumulated stress by labeling it as a routine health step rather than an indicator of mental illness.

Finally, the payoff for such a remediative intervention would be the sustainment of skills, reduction in sick days and medical expenditures, as well as the sustainment of the integrity of the employee's family system. Surely from the economic perspective, remediative intervention makes sense.

References

03OccupationalStressors.pdf. https://info.nicic.gov /virt /sites/info.nicic.gov.virt/files/03OccupationalStr essors.pdf

16-Hour Shifts, 300 Inmates to Watch, and 1 Lonely Son. (2014, December 22). https:// www .themarshallproject.org/2014/12/22/16-hour-shifts-300-inmates-to-watch-and-1-lonely-son

30, J. P. M., & 2016. Forgotten casualties in the war on drugs - The Boston Globe. https:// www.bostong lobe.com/opinion/2016/05/30/forgotten-casualties-war-drugs/NWVfZ2XG 38lFAfFrJ4 P6HK/story.html

ACES Paper for AFC CLE.pdf. https://ubir.buffalo .edu/xmlui/bitstream/handle /10477/25418/ ACES%20Paper%20for%20AFC%20CLE.pdf

Al-Rousan, T., Rubenstein, L., Sieleni, B., Deol, H., & Wallace, R. B. (2017). Inside the nation's largest mental health institution: a prevalence study in a state prison system. *BMC Public Health, 17.* https://doi.org/10.1186/s12889-017-4257-0

Armstrong, G. S., Atkin-Plunk, C. A., & Wells, J. (2015). The Relationship Between Work–Family Conflict, Correctional Officer Job Stress, and Job Satisfaction. *Criminal Justice and Behavior, 42*(10), 1066–1082. https://doi.org/10.1177/0093854815582221

Beating The Odds. http://www.corrections.com/news/article/30096-beating-the-odds

Brain Wars. http://www.pbs.org/wgbh/pages/frontline/traumatic-brain-injury/etc/stories.html

Briere, J., Agee, E., & Dietrich, A. (2016). Cumulative trauma and current posttraumatic stress disorder status in general population and inmate samples. *Psychological Trauma: Theory, Research, Practice and Policy, 8*(4), 439–446. https://doi.org/10.1037/tra0000107

Bureau of Justice Statistics (BJS) - Key Statistic: Total correctional population. https://www.bjs.gov/index.cfm?ty=kfdetail&iid=487

Carroll, H. Going, Going, Gone. http://www.treatmentadvocacycenter.org/going-going-gone

Correctional Officer Duties & Responsibilites | CorrectionalOfficer.org. http://www.correctionalofficer.org/faq/correctional-officer-job-description

Correctional Officer: Education Requirements & Career Info. http://study.com/articles /Correctional_Officer_Educational_Requirements_for_a_Career_in_Corrections.html

Correctional Officer Salaries in the United States | Indeed.com. https://www.indeed. com/salaries/Correctional-Officer-Salaries

Corrections Officer Jobs–What to Expect. http://www.ccu.edu/blogs/cags/2011/10/corrections-officer-jobs-what-to-expect/

Corrections Officers Going To 12 Hour Shifts - Prison Talk. http://www.prisontalk.com /forums/showthread.php?t=537613

Departments Slow to Police Their Own Abusers. (2013, November 24). *The New York Times*. http://www.nytimes.com/projects/2013/police-domestic-abuse/

First Responders and Addiction. (2015, January 28). https://www.morningsiderecovery.com/blog/first-responders-addiction/

Fleischmann, M. H., Strode, P., Broussard, B., & Compton, M. T. (2016). Law enforcement officers' perceptions of and responses to traumatic events: a survey of officers completing Crisis Intervention Team training. *Policing and Society*, *0*(0), 1–8. https://doi.org/10.1080/10439463.2016.1234469

Focus on traumatic childhood helps victims. http://www.postcrescent.com/story/news/investigation

s/2016/05/22/traumatic-childhood-part-one/84649854/

Fox, A. M., Mulvey, P., Katz, C. M., & Shafer, M. S. (2016). Untangling the Relationship Between Mental Health and Homelessness Among a Sample of Arrestees. *Crime & Delinquency, 62*(5), 592–613. https://doi.org/10.1177/0011128713511571

Grammatico, H. (2017). A Phenomenological Study of Correctional Officers' Perceived Emotions on the Job. *Walden Dissertations and Doctoral Studies*. http://scholarworks.waldenu.edu/dissertations/3886

Greene, R. (2016, February 4). From jail to skid row, where "all healing needs are met." *Los Angeles Times*. http://www.latimes.com/opinion/opinion-la/la-ol-starks-los-angeles-homeless-20160203-story.html

Harmon, K., & Harmon, K. Brain Injury Rate 7 Times Greater among U.S. Prisoners. https://www.scientificamerican.com/article/traumatic-brain-injury-prison/

Henning, R. A., Zweber, Z. M., Bizarro, A. M., Bauerle, T., Tubbs, D. C., & Reeves, D. (2017). The Application of Salutogenesis to Correctional Officers in Corrections Settings. In *The Handbook of Salutogenesis* (pp. 247–257). Springer, Cham. https://doi.org/10.1007/978-3-319-04600-6_24

James, L., Todak, N., & Best, S. (2017). The negative impact of prison work on sleep health. *American Journal of Industrial Medicine*, *60*(5), 449–456. https://doi.org/10. 1002/ajim.22714

Konda, S., Tiesman, H., Reichard, A., & Hartley, D. (2013). U.S. Correctional Officers Killed or Injured on the Job. *Corrections Today*, *75*(5), 122–123.

Lurigio, A. J., Belknap, J., Lynch, S., & DeHart, D. (2016). Jail Staff Members' Views on Jailed Women's Mental Health, Trauma, Offending, Rehabilitation, and Reentry. *The Prison Journal*, *96*(1), 79–101. https://doi.org /10.1177/0032 885515605485

MCQ287898.qxd - Sexuality-Masculinity-and-Taint-Management-Among-Firefighters-and-Correctional-Officers-Getting-Down-and-Dirty-With-Americas-Heroes-and-the-Scum-of-Law-Enforcement.pdf. https://www. researchgate .net/profile/ Sarah_Tracy3 /publication/25817 0642_Sexuality_Masculinity_and_Taint_Manag ement_Among_Firefighters_and_Correctional_ Officers_Getting_Down_and_Dirty_With_Amer ica%27s_Heroes_and_the_Scum_of_Law_Enfor cement/links/566882c008ae193b5fa11e6e/Sexua lity-Masc ulinity-and-Taint-Management-Among-Fire fighters-and-Correctional-Officers-Getting-Down-and-Dirty-With-Americas-Heroes-and-the-Scum-of-Law-Enforcement.pdf

Meyer, I. H., Flores, A. R., Stemple, L., Romero, A. P., Wilson, B. D. M., & Herman, J. L. (2017). Incarceration Rates and Traits of Sexual

Minorities in the United States: National Inmate Survey, 2011-2012. *American Journal of Public Health, 107*(2), 267–273. https: //doi.org /10.2105/AJPH.2016.303576

Morel, K., 29, -June, & Said, 2016. (2016, June 28). Alcohol & Cops: The Risks are Real. https:// apbweb.com/alcohol-cops-the-risks-are-real/

Occupational Exposure to Primary and Secondary Trauma in Corrections. http://www.corrections.com/news/article/31682-occupational-exposure-to-primary-and-secondary-trauma-in-corrections

Peters, S. (2017, January 5). Traumatic Brain Injury Associated with Incarceration. https://www.madinamerica.com/2017/01/traumatic-brain-injury-associated-incarceration/

"Prison guards can never be weak": the hidden PTSD crisis in America's jails | US news | The Guardian. https://www.theguardian.com/us-news/2015/may/20/corrections-officers-ptsd-american-prisons

Prisoners on the Eight Rules of Dealing Drugs Behind Bars. http://www.thedaily beast. com/prisoners-on-the-eight-rules-of-dealing-drugs-behind-bars

Scheidell, J. D., Quinn, K., McGorray, S. P., Frueh, B. C., Beharie, N. N., Cottler, L. B., & Khan, M. R. (2017). Childhood Traumatic Exper-iences and the Association with Marijuana and Cocaine Use in Adolescence through Adulthood. *Addiction*

(Abingdon, England). https://doi.org/10.1111/add.13921

Spotlight: Mental health and prisons, the new asylums. https://apps.bostonglobe.com/spotlight/the-desperate-and-the-dead/series/prisons/

Stack, S. J., & Tsoudis, O. (1997). Suicide risk among correctional officers: A logistic regression analysis. *Archives of Suicide Research*, *3*(3), 183–186. https://doi.org/10.1023/A:1009677102357

Stoyanova, R. G., & Harizanova, S. N. (2016). Assessment of the Personal Losses Suffered by Correctional Officers due to Burnout Syndrome. *The International Journal of Occupational and Environmental Medicine*, *7*(1), 33–41.

The Reality of PTSD in Police/Law Enforcement, Emergency Responders, and Custody Services - viewcontent.cgi. http://digital commons.brockport.edu/cgi/viewcontent.cgi?article=1015&context=crj_facpub

The toll of childhood trauma. (2014, June 23). https://ct.counseling.org/2014/06/the-toll-of-childhood-trauma/

The War on Drugs. https://www.aclu.org/issues/mass-incarceration/war-drugs

They drink when they're blue: Stress, peer pressure contribute to police's alcohol culture. (2012, January 15). https://www.dallasnews.com/news/investigations/2012/01/15/they-drink-when-theyre-blue-stress-peer-pressure-contribute-to-polices-alcohol-culture

Traumatic Childhood Experiences Linked to Adult Addictions, Mental Illness and Crime. http://www.lancastercountyreentry.org/item/traumatic-childhood-experiences-and-adult-addictions-mental-illness-crime

Update: Charges dropped against corrections guard. http://www.nevadaappeal.com/news/crime/corrections-guard-arrested-on-domestic-charge-in-carson-city/

Valentine, C., Oehme, K., & Martin, A. (2012). Correctional Officers and Domestic Violence: Experiences and Attitudes. *Journal of Family Violence, 27*(6), 531–545. https://doi.org/10.1007/s10896-012-9448-y

Violanti, J. M., Robinson, C. F., & Shen, R. (2013). Law enforcement suicide: a national analysis. *International Journal of Emergency Mental Health, 15*(4), 289–297.

What's it like being a CO spouse? https://www.correctionsone.com/brandy-alderidge/articles/7205378-Whats-it-like-being-a-CO-spouse/

Working at Illinois Department Of Corrections: 60 Reviews | Indeed.com. https://www.indeed.com/cmp/Illinois-Department-of-Corrections/reviews

Chapter Nine
The Storm

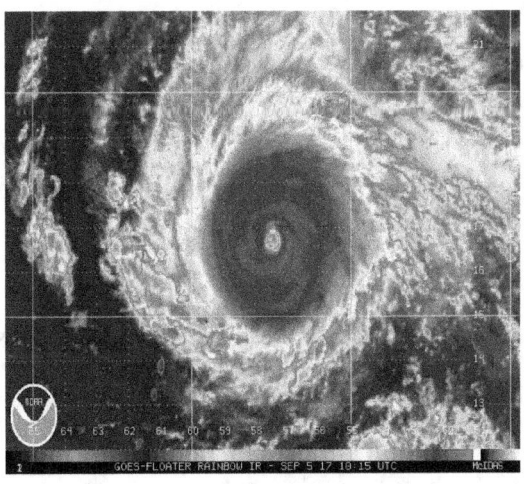

"First, the wind would rumble in the distance like an approaching river, then he would see grass bend, pressed by a great invisible hand. The dull rumble would rise in pitch to a swishing, lashing exultation, causing stalks to lie flat against the ground while the tougher branches of shrubs held themselves up and shrieked their defiance in the gusts. Then the first drops, cold and heavy, would plummet from the sky and burst on the ground."

Jonathan Renshaw, **Dawn of Wonder**

It began in earnest on September 1, 2017 as the remnants of Harvey swept fingers of rain and wind throughout the Bear Creek RV Park in Asheville, North Carolina. This was my day for temporarily transitioning my RV into temporary storage at the campgrounds at the KOA in Swannanoa, N.C. We choose to leave it at this site due to the upcoming weather situation, awaiting our later storing it for the season in the Central Florida region.

After a couple of hesitant first starts, a dire omen of what was to await us, we finally headed in a south easterly direction at approximately 1:00 pm. Our goal was to arrive after two days of travel to our home in Pelican Cove, a beautiful 75-acre gated community located within an environment of beautiful botanical gardens in the south-eastern part of Sarasota County.

Accompanying us were our two rescue dogs and one guest dog respectively named: Chloe, Linus (the bold) and Ollie (neighbor's dog). We lovingly refer to them as the barker, the biter and the pisser. Fortunately, they are wonderful travelers in a car and did well through the random gusts of wind and torrential downbursts of rain.

Our travel plans were to drive for 6 to 7 hours, find a pet friendly hotel/motel and then hunker in for the night. What we hadn't accounted for was that this was the precursor to the Labor Day weekend with the roads filled with traffic as the vacationers proceeded to their choice of holiday location. What we had planned to be a leisurely journey back home for two elderly folks turned into a 14 ½ hour ordeal.

Due to the weather and existing traffic, there was no such pet-friendly hotel/motel to be found. This became a reality as we passed through Stark, Florida headed south towards the I-75 corridor. It was at this point that it became imminently clear that we would have to make it straight to our home in order to be able to secure lodgings for the night.

Thank God, we came upon an open gas station in order to refuel with gas as well as with a large paper cup of high-octane coffee. Around 3:30 a.m. we finally pulled into our designated parking spot in Pelican Cove.

I unloaded the essentials and proceeded to crash for the remainder of the night as well as a good part of the next day. Little did I know what yet lay ahead for us. I remember thinking that old folks such as we weren't meant to travel in such a fashion – that's what the young folk do!

So now we're adjusting to things with the Labor Day event fast approaching. On the Weather Channel, mention was made of yet another storm named Irma forming in the Caribbean. On September 03, 2017, news reports indicated that it was too early to determine what impact Irma will have on the United States mainland.

****

"As she boarded up the windows of her North Naples home, which sits three blocks from the Gulf of Mexico, Gina Fischer left a message for the impending storm. 'Irma go away!' it read in capital letters, painted in red. ("Floridians share their Hurricane Irma stories with CNN - CNN," 2017)

****

Over the following days, the news became increasingly ominous. By September 06, note was made that: "Hurricane Irma, a Category 5 storm rocking winds of 185 mph, battered the north Caribbean on Wednesday and rolled west on what could be a collision course with South Florida over the weekend. If Irma hits the U.S. as a Category 5 storm, it would be just the fourth hurricane of that strength to do so in recorded history. . .

"Bahamas Prime Minister Hubert Minnis ordered the largest evacuation in his nation's history. Michel Magras, senator on the small French-speaking island of St. Barts, sent a text message Wednesday describing the 'monster that passes over us,' 'It is apocalyptic, a lot of damage, a lot of roofs torn off,' he wrote." ("Hurricane Irma: What we know now, where Category 5 storm is headed next," 2017)

By September 07, USA Today noted that: "Hurricane Irma continues to astound and amaze meteorologists with its relentless ferocity. . . Irma had sustained winds of 185 mph for 37 hours, the longest any tropical cyclone around the world has maintained that intensity. The previous record was 24 hours, during Super Typhoon Haiyan in the northwest Pacific in 2013. Irma's 185 mph winds were also the highest on record for a storm in the Atlantic Ocean." ("Hurricane Irma: All the records the storm has broken," 2017)

****

"Antonio Wilson said he is one of only a few residents who rode out the storm in the Icon Brickell towers, which are right on the water in Miami. He decided to stay because he thought he'd be safe.

"'I have some complications with my health and my doctor refused to let me fly out,' Wilson, 35, told CNN on Sunday. 'Because I also have a dog and a cat, I am limited in what I could do. I figured my chances in surviving would be much higher with being in a high rise.'

". . . At this point there isn't much Wilson, an investor, can do. The water is waist-deep around his building, with white-capped waves lapping the foot of the property. 'Everything is flooded,' he said. 'I'm literally stuck.'" ("Floridians share their Hurricane Irma stories with CNN - CNN," 2017)

****

On Friday, September 08, Jack Stevens, General Manager at our Pelican Cove residence issued the following order: "ATTENTION: PELICAN COVE RESIDENTS - PELICAN COVE IS UNDER A MANDATORY EVACUATION NOTICE. SARASOTA COUNTY HAS ISSUED A LEVEL 'A' ORDER. THIS PROMPTS A MANDATORY EVACUATION OF PELICAN COVE TO PROTECT OUR RESIDENTS. Mandatory evacuation issued; shelters open. . . In coordination with the state of Florida, the county has also already opened the following shelter to host evacuees from south Florida:

- Brookside Middle School (pet friendly) 3636 S. Shade Ave., Sarasota.

Around 10:30 am, we hastily packed essential items including bedding, pet food, medications, etc., and headed out to an unfamiliar site in anticipation of a totally unfamiliar shelter experience. We feared for our property and foremost, for our lives as well as those of our pets before the onslaught of this dreaded storm. We've never sheltered before and didn't know the first thing about preparation for this type of experience.

In my mind, I perceived of Irma as being equivalent to a giant Packman chewing up huge expanses of everything in its path – bite by bite. This time was filled with dread as the storm was projected to pass directly through Sarasota accompanied by its full fury.

We made our way to an identified pet-friendly shelter close to us. Now on a typical school day, Brookside Middle School, part of the Sarasota School System nominally receives students. The complex was built to serve multiple functions including that of a shelter facility in times of need. Little did I know that this upcoming calamity would provide me with an opportunity to witness and indirectly participate in the experience of what our first responders, American Red Cross volunteers and assorted citizenry could produce when we came together in times of dire need.

****

"TALLAHASSEE, Fla. - Four-year-old Evan Jackson will be turning 5 on Thursday.

But instead of preparing for a birthday party, his mother, Latoria McKelvey, is bracing herself and her son for Hurricane Irma to rage through Florida. Little Evan has cerebral palsy. He's only able to eat through feeding tubes. And because of low-functioning lungs, he needs breathing treatments several times a day, his mother says.

"When she heard about the Department of Health's special needs shelter stationed at Florida High School, she was relieved. She was one of the first to settle there, bright and early when it opened Saturday morning.

"'(I was) slightly panicked because I didn't know where I was going to go or what I was going to do,' she said, calmly rocking Evan under his favorite Mickey Mouse blanket, in one of the several beds on the floor of the school's pristine gymnasium." ("Floridians share their Hurricane Irma stories with CNN - CNN," 2017)

****

Now I must fess up and tell you that this was a scary experience at times for me, at other times it was an adventure. From my wife's perspective, it was a nightmare. She was of the mind that our pets got to shelter with us. She had a hard time dealing with their being placed in a kennel in a separate building.

Throughout this book, I chose to focus upon the deleterious effects of prolonged exposure to stress on our first responder's mental health and physical wellness. Now it came to me, in a moment of clarity, that I could see them collectively at their best, responding to the uncertainty of the calamity that was predicted to be rapidly heading toward us.

A little background about the American National Red Cross, as it was called at the time, to begin this discourse. It was created in Washington, D.C. on May 21, 1881, by Clara Barton who became its first president. Sarah led one of the group's first major relief efforts, a response to the September 4–6, 1881 Great Fire in the Thumb Region of Michigan where over 5,000 people were left homeless.

The American Red Cross (ARC) currently consists of a nationwide network of more than 650 chapters and 36 blood service regions. "Approximately 500,000 Red Cross volunteers, including FemaCorps and AmeriCorps members, and 30,000 employees annually mobilize relief to people affected by more than 67,000 disasters, train almost 12 million people in necessary medical skills and exchange more than a million emergency messages for U.S. military service personnel and their family members.

". . . In addition to disaster relief, the ARC also "provides emergency and non-emergency services to the United States military. The most notable service is emergency family communications, where families can contact the Red Cross to send important family messages (such as a death in the family, or new birth)." ("American Red Cross," 2017)

****

"The gas station's slow-moving line stretched to nearly 20 cars, drivers desperate to top off tanks before the storm blows through the capital. Saturday afternoon, it was one of the only gas stations in sight with a digital sign that was not blank. About 6 miles north, hundreds hunkered down at Chiles High School, which the Red Cross has turned into a shelter.

"Inside, volunteers stood at the entrance handing out neatly folded donated clothes. In the gymnasium, dozens of air mattresses and blankets were spread out. Dozens filed in, some stopping for an extra shirt at the donation table, others carrying large bulk boxes of Cheetos and Chips Ahoy.

". . . Debbie Mann, a local Red Cross volunteer, was helping manage the shelter. She said Saturday it was at maximum capacity, with more than 500 people checked in. 'It's a safe haven. It's some place for the families to be together and weather out this storm together,' said Mann. 'that's the most important thing — is family. Everything else is replaceable.'" ("Fleeing Hurricane Irma: A family with special needs, and a survivor of Katrina, Harvey," 2017)

****

By Thursday, September 09, Fox News reported that: "A hurricane-force wind gust was recorded in the Florida Keys late Saturday night -- the first sign of deadly Hurricane Irma's impending landfall on the U.S. mainland. The weather service said the Smith Shoal Light station recorded a 74-mph wind gust on Saturday night, the Associated Press reported. Meanwhile, the center of Irma was headed toward the Keys with sustained winds of 120 mph.

"The edge of Hurricane Irma kicked up surf, whipped up palm trees and spun up at least one confirmed tornado as it approached landfall in Florida Saturday evening. Irma had been downgraded to a Category 3 storm as it raked the coast of Cuba Saturday morning, but it was expected to get its strength back over the ultra-toasty Florida Straits and hit the peninsula Sunday morning as a dangerous Category 4 storm." ("Hurricane Irma: What we know now, where Category 5 storm is headed next,")

On Friday, September 10th Hurricane Irma wreaked: "havoc in Florida, its floodwaters have inundated the streets of Miami, making the city completely unrecognizable. The hurricane, now downgraded to a Category 2 storm, had wind speeds of 130 mph while a Category 3 when it pounded palm trees along Brickell Ave. in the city's downtown financial area.

"Videos on social media show a battered South Beach as floodwaters rushed through streets, entered businesses and residences. Earlier, Irma's ferocious winds caused a crane to snap. A second tower crane has also collapsed into a building that was under construction, Miami City Manager Daniel Alfonso said.

"Meteorologists have urged the public to not go outside due to storm surges that could rise rapidly. . . . More than 2 million Floridians have lost power, and of the 845,000 plus Florida Power & Light customers are in Miami-Dade County, the utility company, which serves South Florida, reported.

"Emergency services were suspended until winds slow down to less than 40 mph. An 8 p.m. curfew has been imposed for Miami over the next two nights, and no one is allowed out on the streets until they are cleared, Miami Beach officials said. Thousands of families have fled to shelters, even as others remained home to ride out the storm, despite mandatory evacuation in their respective counties." ("1 sec 8," 2017)

****

"While spending the night in a place she didn't know, two-and-a-half-year-old Mya fell asleep nestled on her father's back. 'She didn't want to leave her daddy's side, so she fell asleep on it,' said Melissa Tuccio. Tuccio, along with her boyfriend Chris McInerney and their five children, live in San Carlos Park, Florida, but have been staying at a shelter in nearby Estero since Thursday.

"'We have switched from food donations from the Red Cross to military meals,' Tuccio told CNN on Sunday morning. Available cots there are sparse. Tuccio said her family gave up one of their beds this weekend to a veteran who is on oxygen.

"There is coffee, though. The line for a warm cup of joe stretched about 20 to 30 people deep, snaking down the shelter's hallway. The family isn't sure how long they will be in the shelter. They've been asked to stay put at least until Monday, she said." ("Floridians share their Hurricane Irma stories with CNN - CNN," 2017)

****

Frankly, on Friday, September 08 it began as a mad house scenario as multitudes of people emerged on Brookside Middle School to register both themselves and their beloved pets. As part of the process, the pets were to be secured in a separate room in crates that the owners were expected to have accompanying them.

We had no such crate being totally ignorant of the process and the kindly, understanding Red Cross volunteer offered us a large one that could be used to house all three small dogs so that they could remain together. The barking and whining of the accumulated dogs reached a crescendo that hurt the ears and dulled the other senses. Later, the smells would add to the impact.

We were told that they could be visited, taken outside and comforted, fed, etc., up until the moment of imminent danger at which point, the doors would be locked and secured. Cats were secured in another room. It was quite pathetic to see people separated from their animals as though this might be the last time they might see them again.

As for us frightened humans, the long registration line was the beginning of the process. Parking was also an issue as the lines of cars quickly jammed up to the entrance to the school. Later I learned that a bus that was transporting older residents of a nursing home removed individuals, one at a time, through a lift system as well as individually unloading their wheelchairs, bottles of oxygen etc. Some of the impatient drivers were becoming short-tempered until Sarasota police and Sherriff personnel stepped in to establish 'law and order.'

On the registration line in the massive school cafeteria, hundreds of people awaited to sign in and to be designated a square of about 3 by 3 feet to await their assigned location for the upcoming ordeal. They toted with them their belongings filling the space they were allocated quite rapidly. All languages were spoken with Spanish being prominent among them.

People were clearly frightened of the impending unknown. One small tv set was tuned into the Weather Channel in the cafeteria announcing the ominous path of the threatening storm. People were clustered around it in disbelief of the steamroller that was headed our way.

The first call for a dinner meal took place around 5:00 with a long conga style line immediately forming and then snaking throughout the cafeteria space. Now I'm unsure if what we were fed was chicken sticks or fish sticks with Mac and cheese. Whatever it was, it was warm and appreciated. The American Red Cross volunteers maintained their calm and collected state in the midst of this seeming calamity that included families being inadvertently separated from each other. Elderly persons became lost from their group and were unable to provide clarity other than a name. But then gradually, calm replaced fear as the structure for the sheltering plan began to slowly emerge.

I approached a Red Cross official to inquire where the First Aid Station was located. Upon finding it, I provided a card and introduced myself as an available psychologist if and when there was a need for my assistance. Jokingly, one of the attending nurses said that she could use an appointment right now.

Back to the registration area, my wife and I were assigned to the school gym area where we inhabited two assigned blue-taped squares that were approximately 3 by 3 feet. No tv or other forms of communication were available although a loudspeaker system permitted announcements as the occasion required. Gradually, the cafeteria was cleared as people went to their designated locations.

Upon returning to the gym, we were informed that it could not withstand the expected hurricane winds and that we were to be assigned to a classroom instead. A police officer directed us to our designated area. In our classroom were 18 members of an extended Argentinian family with a number of them US citizens and others visiting Miami from Buenos Aires only to flee north due to the upcoming storm. A few like ourselves were elderly. Some spoke both English and Spanish, others did not. A few were rambunctious kids. Another elderly couple as well as ourselves comprised the 22 persons assigned to Building 04, Room 110.

A large tv was on the wall but no connection was available. Only later was a computer knowledgeable member of the Argentinian family able to connect it to his computer so we could follow the storm and entertain ourselves by watching a Smurf movie. I thought, geez, this might turn out to be fun rather that the horrible experience we all expected!

Not far behind us was stationed an EMT unit that was later joined by two National Guard transport trucks. From time to time, the EMT's wheeled out persons in need of medical assistance that couldn't be provided on the site. I didn't initially realize that this went on throughout the night after lights out at 10 and lockdown that occurred at 11 pm.

Up until that time, we were free to visit, provide comfort and attend to our pets, receive storm updates on the little TV in the cafeteria and have a hot meal around dinner time with hundreds of others standing on the dreaded lines once again. Now mind you, it wasn't the Ritz, but it sure beat the alternatives.

****

"The breakfast table was in the school's cafeteria, jampacked with hungry evacuees who tiptoed around the sleeping bags scattered all over the floor. 'They didn't have to do this for us, this is really nice of them,' said an evacuee from Indian Rocks Beach, Florida.

"The cafeteria is the nerve center of the evacuation complex. It's has most of the TVs, and people were glued to CNN and the local stations and their wall-to-wall coverage of the hurricane. It's also where the people who were trying to keep their minds off the storm gathered. A couple of men played chess; most were gathered in conversation; many continued to catch some sleep.

"Throughout it all, there was little chaos. People seem resigned to the situation and were doing their best to weather the storm. The kids were being kids, running the halls and keeping parents on their toes. Local volunteers were busy keeping things in order, cleaning up as best they could and emptying garbage cans to try and keep ahead of the game hygienically.

"Police took one man back to his vehicle to get rid of the gun he thought he'd be able to bring into the shelter. He received a resounding no and a lecture from an officer for being so foolish.

"Otherwise, all was calm. But the elephant was never far from the room. After all, no one would be here but for the impending storm. ("In Florida shelter, exhausted people wait out Hurricane Irma," 2017)

****

One of the members of the Argentinian family brought out a cluster of light bulbs the type of which I've never seen before. Each one was apparently battery powered and a few were hung from the ceiling in the event the power went out or to give us some semblance of lighting if necessary.

We were alerted through the speaker system and visiting Red Cross representative as to recommended toilet procedures. The yellow stuff accumulates, the other stuff gets flushed through using water we are to save in designated buckets for that specific purpose. And so, gradually we all settled in for the night dressed in the same garment we were in during the day of arrival. In fact, we stayed in the same clothes until the experience ended on the following Monday, four days later.

The building we were in insulated us from the sounds of the accumulating storm although we could see the small palm trees beginning to wave as well as the rain occasionally hitting the pavement. With lights-out, everything became surreal.

Bodies trying to sleep here and there, some on air-mattresses, some on pads and others on blankets laid on the tile floor. Kids not yet ready to bed-down looking at their I-pads. People making their way to the restrooms. Finally, quiet!

The next morning awakening to realize that we were still alive. The signs remained ominous as Irma was projected to brutalize Cuba and then head straight for Miami sweeping upward through the center of Florida consuming the entire state. I envisioned a giant Packman gobbling up the entire peninsula.

The storm, we were told, extended well over 400 miles extending over the entire breadth of the state with winds projected at upwards of 130 to 140mph. What a nightmare was heading our way!

At around 6:30 am we took our pets out for their morning relief feeding them at 7:00. We spent time giving them touch-care to alleviate the confinement of the kennel. As an aside, rescue dogs, which ours were, generally don't do well in confinement of this type. Fortunately, our pets seemed to adapt to the circumstances, settling in accordingly.

****

"Life waits for no one and no storm, as two expectant mothers learned during Hurricane Irma. On Sunday, a pregnant human and a pregnant dog both went into labor at the same storm shelter in Brooksville, Florida. According to WKPG, as Irma raged outside the two moms prepared to give birth at D.S. Parrott Middle School, a designated shelter open to not just animals lovers, but their pets as well.

"The human mom, seven and half month pregnant, was rushed to a nearby hospital to give birth shortly after her contractions started. Both mom and baby are doing well.

"Chyanne the 3-year-old husky Siberian husky mix, who went into labor around the same time, stayed at the shelter to deliver her pups, giving birth seven days past her due date. She was helped through the miracle of life by belly rubs from her owner and the care of Brent Gaustad, the principal at D.S. Parrott Middle School. Animal services was also on site to assist.

"Amidst the chaos of Irma, these dual births were a welcome ray of celebration for Gaustad and others at the shelter. The principal sees these new arrivals as "unique" and "wonderful" breaks to a stressful situation. ("Hurricane Irma: Pregnant Woman and Dog Go Into Labor at Florida Hurricane Shelter," 2017)

****

So here we are on Sunday the 10th awaiting the arrival of the dreaded storm. We had our last hot meal the evening before and were provided with a bag of stuff from the Red Cross. Mine included the following: Smucker's Uncrustables – peanut butter & grape jelly sandwich; Dick & Jane Educational Snacks; Cinnamon Toast Crunch – Real Cinnamon & Sugar in Every Delicious Bite.

At 1:30 pm that Sunday the announcement came that we were now on lockdown as the effects of the storm were rapidly approaching us. The projected path of the storm shifted rapidly with Miami alleged to be entirely under water and landfall now expected to shift to and now hit Naples, a short distance south from us.

At around 3:30 pm, the power went out in our building. We later found out it was the only one to do so. On the prior evening, a faucet in the men's room became stuck flooding the room thereby making it unavailable and unsanitary. Four adjoining classrooms connected via hallways with only one bathroom available. In spite of these obstacles, we kept our cool.

During the evening, an elderly woman appearing dazed and confused wandered into our room, apparently becoming lost in the hallway maze. She was headed for the exit door in an attempt to leave the building. I approached her asking her name. She responded with 'Phyllis" and I asked her if she would like my help in finding her way back. She responded with a yes and I walked with her to the varied rooms until finally, when we visited the final classroom, someone claimed her.

By Saturday, September 11, Hurricane Irma "reached Naples with a terrifying force. The Naples

Municipal Airport recorded a wind gust of 142 mph – the highest reported in Florida.

"Naples Mayor Bill Barnett, who was also the city's mayor during Hurricanes Charley and Wilma in 2004 and 2005, said the city 'took a real hard hit.' But as for the 'good news,' he pointed to the storm surge.

"Storm surge here was predicted to be anywhere between 12 and 18 feet. And we really dodged that. We had minimal, minimal storm surge. Still have a lot of water though, and there are couple neighborhoods we can't even get into, Barnett told 'CBS This Morning' Monday, as he was out assessing the damage.

"Luckily and thankfully so far not a lot of structural damage. I will tell you that there are road blocks. There's flooding. There is a neighborhood – that are badly flooded. I'm looking at a tree right now that's on top of a transformer box, so Florida Power & Light is going to have a massive, massive, massive job, not just in Naples but all across the state as you know," Barnett said. The storm knocked out power to more than 6.5 million Florida residents.

"The only structural damage down there was it blew the roof off of a – we have a fire station there but it's only manned for the airports. So nobody hurt.

And if that's the worst, we can live with it for sure," Barnett added.

****

"Like many during Hurricane Hermine last year, McKelvey lost power in her Blountstown home for five days. 'I didn't want to take that chance,' she said about Hurricane Irma. 'Especially with him being totally dependent on the feeding pump.' The shelter has generators and offers bedding and staffed nurses for people who need extra care like Evan, or those who are oxygen-dependent or wheelchair-bound.

"Like McKelvey, this isn't Zonia Thompson's first hurricane either. This is her third time being displaced. Twelve years ago, Thompson and her then-3-month-old daughter Samyra Bickham fled Louisiana because of Hurricane Katrina. They lost everything then.

"Most recently, Hurricane Harvey flooded her newly rented home in Houston. She had just moved there two months ago for a new welding job. But that new life was quickly overturned when Harvey ravaged through Houston and destroyed hundreds of homes, including hers.

"Thompson and Samyra, now 12, came to Miami to escape Harvey . . But Irma forced them to pick up and leave — again. . . 'It's been an ongoing struggle,' said Thompson. "It's like I'm literally running from storms."

"Thompson and her family are Louisiana-bound but stopped for a break and some food at a Shell gas station in Tallahassee. Her two restless, toddler-aged grandchildren laughed and ran around an empty parking spot with her son-in-law, stretching their legs after a 12-hour drive. 'I just keep losing houses and everything I've worked for.' Thompson said, blankly staring into the distance through sunglasses." ("Fleeing Hurricane Irma: A family with special needs, and a survivor of Katrina, Harvey," 2017)

****

Hurricane Irma weakened to a tropical storm Monday, but the extreme weather has lashed nearly every part of Florida. Irma is blamed for the worst storm sure flooding ever recorded in cities like Jacksonville. Irma is now moving north, dumping huge amounts of rain in Alabama, Georgia, and South Carolina.

Barnett said he knows it's going to be an expensive cleanup, but "so far I haven't heard of any injuries or ... loss of lives, and so I'm really pleased about that." (11, 2017, & Pm,)

I later learned that many of those from the nursing homes became lost and that pictures were taken of them and circulated to identify the group they were affiliated with. This adaptive step clearly helped to return to confused back to their safe harbor. Clearly, an emerging supportive community of first responders and Red Cross volunteers came into rapid existence in the shelter seeing to the needs of each of the occupants in a caring and compassionate way.

Finally, on Monday morning after a scary, anxious ridden night (9/12/17) we were informed that the danger had passed us and was now headed north to release its damage on the central and western coast of Florida. We in the assigned room said farewell to each other and began packing out our belongings. As suddenly as it occurred, it was over. People left in an orderly fashion returning to their homes accordingly. I exchanged cards with those I met asking them to stay in touch.

Taking a look at this in a broader perspective, things came together as they were meant to be. Our first responders were at the core of this conflagration of people from all walks of life. They quietly, efficiently and professionally saw to the physical needs of those who required it. They maintained the structure necessary for this hastily concocted community to function well within the context of a potential natural disaster.

The Brookside Middle School Principal made timely and frequent announcements over the loudspeaker system to keep the community informed of matters of concern. Nurses and doctors manned the clinic to see to the medical needs that could be met at the shelter. Those with needs that extended beyond existing resources were taken by EMT personnel to a designated site that could assist them.

The presence of police and sheriff personnel served to maintain order and block hysteria from breaking through the fear so many had as to what was soon to be upon us. The national guard personnel stood at the ready to transport large numbers of people if the need arose. The Red Cross volunteers fed us, protected and saw to our pets, visited us in our designated rooms to answer questions and engaged in a myriad of activities throughout our shelter experience. They did all this leaving their families behind to see to the needs of this newly developed community of strangers.

Upon returning to Pelican Cove, I later learned of others who chose to remain, rather than utilize shelter facilities. My neighbor, M. K., shared her story with me.

****

"For a few days before the upcoming storm, I was caring for a close family friend, who was dying of cancer. We were aware of sign-up locations for adult persons with special medical needs.

I filled out the application for my friend and sent it in expecting him to be picked up by a van prior to the arrival of the storm. That evening, he was 'sundowning' and becoming thoroughly confused.

"His caregivers and I got all of his stuff together but by noon, the van hadn't arrived and we were without power with the temperature rising to around 90 degrees. We took him to the designated shelter and they wouldn't take him. We called 911 and the EMT's were able to make it past the fallen trees blocking the roadway. They were thorough in gathering information on his condition such as that related to his feeding tube.

Four of them carefully took him down from our second-floor condo. They were wonderful! My friend was dazed, not understanding why they were taking him to Sarasota Memorial Hospital. Without their assistance, I don't think he could have made it through that day. 2017"

****

For their personal sacrifice, our first responders, ARC volunteers and all who supported the effort deserve our unwavering appreciation. From my perspective, they also deserve to know that there is an effective way to release the effects of cumulative stress that alters their mental and physical well-being over time.

My mission has been to end the ongoing nightmare of PTSD among our active duty and veteran communities. To this I whole heartedly add the community of first responders. They surely deserve the blessing of intact body, mind and soul as they sacrifice to keep us safe and secure.

References

1 sec 8. http://www.ora.tv/homepage /2016/8 /29/5?break_aspect_ratio=true

11, C. N. S., 2017, & Pm, 2:00. Hurricane Irma: Naples, Florida mayor says city "dodged" storm surge predictions. https://www .cbsnews.com/news /hurricane-irma-naples-florida-mayor-bill-barnett-damage/

American Red Cross. (2017, September 15). In *Wikipedia*. https://en.wikipedia.org/w/index.php?title=American_Red_Cross&oldid=800700790

Fleeing Hurricane Irma: A family with special needs, and a survivor of Katrina, Harvey. https://www.usatoday.com/story/news/nation-now/2017/09/09/fleeing-hurricane-irma-special-needs-family-and-survivor-katrina-and-harvey/650499001/

Floridians share their Hurricane Irma stories with CNN - CNN. http://www.cnn.com/2017/09/10/us/hurricane-irma-text-whatsapp-messages-trnd/index.html

Hurricane Irma: All the records the storm has broken. https://www.usatoday.com/story/weather/2017/09/07/all-records-hurricane-irma-has-already-broken/642948001/

Hurricane Irma: Pregnant Woman and Dog Go Into Labor at Florida Hurricane Shelter. http://people.com/pets/hurricane-irma-human-and-dog-mom-labor-florida-shelter/

Hurricane Irma: What we know now, where Cate-gory 5 storm is headed next. https://www.usatoday.com/story/news/nation/2017/09/06/hurricane-irma-what-we-know-now-and-where-its-headed-next/636682001/

In Florida shelter, exhausted people wait out Hurricane Irma. http://www.catholicnews.com/services

/englishnews/2017/in-florida-shelter-exhausted-people-wait-out-hurricane-irma.cfm

Chapter Ten

THE HEALING SOUND

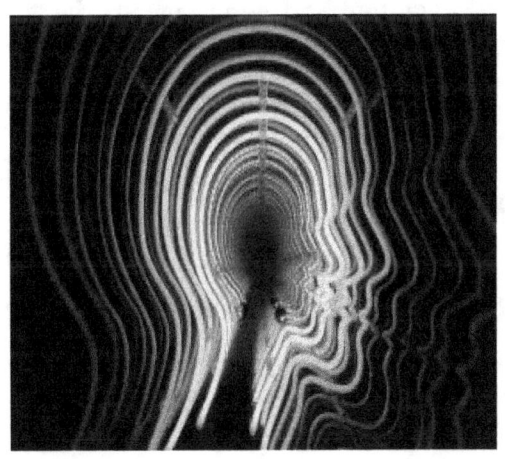

"Music sets up a certain vibration
which unquestionably results in a physical
reaction. Eventually the proper vibration for
every person will be found and utilized."

George Gershwin

"Loud sounds can elevate our stress levels, create imbalances in our nervous system, lower our immunity and, in extreme cases, cause hearing loss. When we are stressed, our whole relationship to sound changes, and regular everyday sounds can become magnified and contribute to the feedback cycle of the stress, amplifying it even more." (Lee, 2012)

Much of the current work on the healing properties of sound is based on the early 70's research of biophysicist, Dr. Gerald Oster. Oster, who showed that when a tone is played in one ear and a slightly different tone is played in the other ear, the difference causes the brain to perceive a third internal tone called a binaural beat." (Wagner 2013)

In the realm of healing techniques, sound has been used for thousands of years, yet it's also on the frontiers of modern neuroscience. What's important for you to know in this discussion is that the properly set binaural beat that resonates with an emotional target is the means through which we can eliminate the emotional component of the PTSD condition. We now have the means to tune into the 'proper vibration' for each person and to use that frequency to resonate with selected trauma targets.

Physicists and acoustic engineers tend to discuss sound pressure levels in terms of frequencies, partly because this is how our ears interpret sound. What we experience as a 'higher pitch' or 'lower pitch' are pressure vibrations having higher or lower numbers of cycles per second. This is also an important element in properly setting therapeutic sound levels to create a transformative opportunity.

Binaural beats are created by sounds of slightly differing frequency in each ear and the brain perceiving of them as one. This kind of neuromodulated sound has been proposed to induce relaxation, meditation, creativity and other desirable mental states. This effect was discovered initially in 1839 by Heinrich Wilhelm Dove, with greater public awareness emerging in the late 20th century. (Ashton, 2010)

"There have been a number of unsubstantiated claims regarding binaural beats, including that they may help people memorize and learn, stop smoking, help with dieting, and improve athletic performance.

While these claims may or may not be valid, we believe that the sensation of binaural beats originates in a part of the brain stem that appears to be related to the brain's ability to locate the sources of sounds in three dimensions and to track moving sounds." ("Triggers & Flashbacks" 2001)

One hundred and thirty-four years after Dove's original discovery, Gerald Oster published an article in *Scientific American* titled, "Auditory Beats in the Brain." (Oster, 1973) In particular, Oster saw binaural beats as a powerful tool for brain research that focused on questions such as how animals locate sounds in their three-dimensional environment.

Oster also considered binaural beats to be a potentially useful medical tool. He believed that this tool could be used not only for finding and assessing auditory impairments, but also for more general neurological conditions because binaural beats involve different neurological pathways than ordinary auditory processing." (Barr, Mullin, & Herbert, 1977)

At this point in our discussion, let me introduce you to the Bio-Acoustical Utilization Device (BAUD) created with basic protocols by Dr. Frank Lawlis and his son, T Frank Lawlis. The Bio-Acoustical Utilization Device (BAUD) is a FDA class 2 accessory medical device designed to enhance brain plasticity in biofeedback programs. The device creates independent square sound waves from 39 to

362 Hz. that are heard separately in the left and right ears.

Dr. Lawlis perceives that the underlying acoustical physics entrain the general EEG ranges by creating a third tone [the beat frequency] from the interference ratios between the two frequencies (Lawlis. 2009) It is thus purported to influence brain functioning at an unconscious level and perceived emotional functioning at the conscious level. Note: I personally perceive that the effects of the BAUD are not due to an entrainment process but rather, to an interruption of the memory reconsolidation process.

RESET Therapy is the treatment process utilizing the BAUD and its protocols that interfere with targeted trauma memories. It blocks repeated restoration after it is selectively lit up in the emotional part of the brain through the patient's intentional focus. I use the term "target" in RESET Therapy and suggest to my patient that we are going to turn off the 'switch' in the brain that produces the PTSD symptoms (Lindenfeld & Bruursema, 2015)

Experientially, I've learned that my patients tend to fall into one of three groups. The first cluster experiences immediate relief ranging from partial to complete reduction of the targeted symptom. The second group notices a slight change initially that seems to build over the course of 24 hours. The third group, a minority, experiences no change at all.

I ask the patient to inform me of their response to the RESET Therapy the next day by phone, text or e-mail so that I can plan accordingly for our next scheduled session. With the first and second group, I proceed with full intervention when the next appointment occurs.

With the third group, I seek to clarify whether the target was fully activated. Often, I find that the patient doesn't understand what I mean by this due to a variety of factors. In extreme circumstances, I have found a dissociative disconnect that blocks the spontaneous merging of material from the body and the mind.

When this disconnect is present, alternative interventions such as ART (Accelerated Resolution Therapy) can often break through the mind/body blockage, permitting reconsideration of the use of RESET Therapy once again (The Rosenzweig Center for Rapid Recovery; http://accelerated-resolution therapy.com/web/how-art-works/ n.d.)

I've not run into a situation where it was not possible to find a creative way through the psychic wall, although I can imagine that this could occur. When the next full intervention session occurs, the patient is asked to "run the script" internally for a full 15 to 20 minutes. More often than not, the patient reports that his/her inner mind took over from the script and ran its own agenda of nightmares, flashbacks, etc. When it occurs, I encourage this shift to the inner mind from the patient's conscious control efforts.

During the 'tuning in' trial and the full 15 to 20-minute treatment session, I remain busy. I'm carefully observing body signals, changes in breathing patterns and facial expressions while recording my observations within the context of the treatment.

One of my older patients came up with an awareness that her unconscious mind liked what was happening. She said: "Mikey likes it," referring to an old cereal ad that most of you probably haven't heard of. However, I use this phrase to clarify the 'letting-go' process, particularly for those who struggle to maintain whatever existing control they perceive they still have.

Paradoxically, after 5 minutes or so, the annoying sound is reported by many to become increasingly comfortable. When asked later what had occurred, the patient typically notes a sort of dissolving or fading effect of the targeted material.

When asked after the treatment to discuss the target, the patient typically says something to the effect that he/she can recall with more clarity what happened at the time of the original incident but that the uncomfortable emotional component was gone. It is typically at this point that the patient's trauma can be conveyed verbally, fully and completely, rather than in the fragments that predominated before treatment.

Following the full intervention session, I ask the patient to remain skeptical to the RESET experience and, as noted earlier, to call me 24 hours later to report any changes that may have occurred. Often, I receive positive feedback such as the patient experiencing a full night's sleep, none of the previous cold sweats at night, no anger outbursts at loved ones, no horrible flashbacks.

It still gets to me at an emotional level when I hear this. I feel as though I've facilitated someone's return from the brink. When you get to experience this phenomenon personally, it's like nothing else you've encountered before. You begin to anticipate the excitement of what this day and the days to come will bring as you shift back to a growth mode leaving the 'protect and defend' one behind.

This is the point that insight begins to flow to your mind, permitting a full and complete comprehension of the targeted trauma experience. After the fear switch has been flipped off, you have the opportunity to become the person you were before the trauma encounter.

Finally, when this procedure is provided carefully by an adequately trained and certified therapist, your nightmares and flashbacks are finally, completely and permanently gone! Your transformative experience removes the entrapped poison, permitting you to personally experience the elation and joy of participation in this process. This becomes enhanced even further when your 'thousand-yard stare' instantly disappears and is replaced by a look of wonderment. I assure you, this is a moment that you will never forget.

If we were to look at the RESET process through an fMRI, specific areas deep within the brain such as the amygdala would appear to be activated (flared) and other brain areas such as the speech center located in the left hemisphere would be shut down, going off line when the trauma was triggered. The area that is associated with making complex decisions in the prefrontal lobes referred to as 'executive functioning' also goes off line when the trauma is reactivated. (Bomyea, Risbrough, & Lang, 2012).

Perhaps this pattern is the reason that talking to someone in the depths of their PTSD despair hardly ever does anything but frustrate the speaker, whose words can't be fully received by the supposed listener. Also, perhaps this is why the person with PTSD seems dumfounded by tasks that he/she was previously well able to manage. (Lanius et al., 2004)

Another area located in the visual cortex is called Brodmann's Area 19. (Lanius et al., 2004) This part of the brain receives images conveyed from the eyes and supports feature extraction, shape recognition, visual attention, and multimodal integration.

Unfortunately, with the onset of PTSD, it also triggers a rekindling visual aspect of trauma, often referred to as flashbacks. Other senses such as smell, sound and visceral sensations also are likely to be reactivated in flashbacks (Bomyea et al., 2012). Consequently, I have come to refer to the following pattern of limbic system activation, speech inhibition, cognitive inhibition, and in some cases, flashbacks as the **Neuronal Model of PTSD.**

To reiterate, when an individual is traumatized as evidenced in fMRI studies, the following happens; The connection to the prefrontal cortex shuts down, leading to a decline in the ability to understand and a diminishment in the executive functioning that previously existed.

Secondly, the speech centers located in the left hemisphere of the brain suffers the same fate, with the PTSD sufferer being left with an ability to address only fragments of the trauma. This makes it difficult for him/her to fully articulate what happened in the first place. It also filters the ability to hear from others in a complete and meaningful way (Burke, 2008).

The person becomes unable to fully express what has occurred. Furthermore, he/she becomes unable to benefit from what others say. Next, the Limbic System becomes over activated, perpetuating the 'fight, flight or freeze' instinctual response. Finally, Brodmann's Area 19 rekindles visual and other sensory aspects of trauma referred to as flashbacks.

You have now been introduced to this incredibly effective treatment that I call RESET Therapy that can place PTSD into full and total remission. Others are trying to connect with specific areas of the brain, such as the Limbic System, by placing electrodes in the brain through invasive surgical procedures. Contrast that approach with this non-invasive and safe form of intervention, which is relatively free from side effects.

More often than not, when only one target is involved, it is necessary for the patient to go through this unique ordeal only one time in non-complex Post-Traumatic Stress Disorder. After experiencing rapid relief from this initial encounter, my patients tell me that they would have little hesitation to engage in the process again if a new target surfaces, and to do this as often as required to fully clear out any remaining remnants of trauma.

At this point, let me introduce you to Greg Para, the Courts Assisting Veterans Coordinator at 12th Judicial Circuit Court, which covers three Florida counties including Sarasota, Manatee and DeSoto. Diagnosed with anxiety disorder after his 2011-2012 tour of Afghanistan, Greg still has difficulty when it comes to hypervigilance.

He was approached as a potential referral source for combat veterans with PTSD for a current research project being conducted in the greater Sarasota,

Florida region. The outcome of this effort would result in the compiling of a database for submission into a scientific journal documenting the amazing effects of RESET Therapy in the remediation of PTSD symptomology. Greg decided to volunteer himself first so might be able to give his veterans a fair assessment of whether RESET Therapy would work for him or not.

****

"'Like anyone who suffers from anything, you'll try anything to get relief', says Para. 'And I told (Lindenfeld) I'd do it first.' After four sessions with the RESET headphones, Para was a convert. 'The nightmares weren't the only things that disappeared.'

"'Driving, for me, was an exhausting event, constantly scanning the horizon, looking at packages and things on the side of the road, dealing with people who cut in and out without using their blinkers. I'm telling you, I would get short of breath, my heartbeat would get up to 140, it was just nuts,' he says. 'That's why I didn't go to work for the first six months after I got back (from Afghanistan).

> "RESET allowed me to do something (driving) that, when I thought about it, would get me to a 10 on the anxiety chart. Now I can't get above a 3, even if I tried."

****

I've included an example of results forthcoming from RESET Therapy as I've alluded to its potential to remediate PTSD and compassion fatigue throughout this book. While outside of the military it may be called 'Compassion Fatigue" but by my account, it's the same thing.

We can and must utilize new scientific breakthroughs to sustain the skills and capability of our essential personnel. I believe that RESET Therapy will be one of many such tools available to us to sustain the quality of life of our first responders.

Reference List:

Arem, K. The Future of Sound Therapy. *Music as Medicine*. Informational. http://gaearth.com/sound-as-medicine/the-future-of-sound-therapy/

Ashton, N. (2010, November 8). Discovery Of Binaural Beats. *Binaural Blog*. http:// www.binauralblog.com/?p=6

Barr, D. F., Mullin, T. A., & Herbert, P. S. (1977). Application of binaural beat phenomenon with aphasic patients. *Archives of Otolar-yngology (Chicago, Ill.: 1960), 103*(4), 192–194.

Bomyea, J., Risbrough, V., & Lang, A. J. (2012). A consideration of select pre-trauma factors as key vulnerabilities in PTSD. *Clinical Psychology Review, 32*(7), 630–641. http://doi.org/ 10.1016/j.cpr.2012.06.008

Burke, T. K. (2008). *How Trauma Impacts the Brain.* Informational presented at the Rachel's Vineyard Retreat, Canada. http://www.rachels vineyard.org /Downloads/Canada%20 Conference%2008/TextOfBrainPP.pdf

Lanius, R. A., Williamson, P. C., Densmore, M., Boksman, K., Neufeld, R. W., Gati, J. S., & Menon, R. S. (2004). The Nature of Trau-matic Memories: A 4-T fMRI Functional Connectivity Analysis. *American Journal of Psychiatry, 161*(1), 36–44. http://doi.org /10.1176/appi .ajp.161.1.36

Lawlis, F. *An international clinical study of the sonic disruption of sympathetic arousal princip-le as designed in the BAUD device.* Lewisville, TX: Lawlis-Peavey PNP Center. http://www .baud energetics.com/images/ study %20for %20sonic%20disruptor%20 in%20int' l%20study.pdf

Lee, J. (2012, July 17). Noise and Stress – How Environmental Noise Levels Can Spike Your Stress Load. *Choose Help.* Informat-ional. http://www.choosehelp. com/topics /stress-burnout/noise-and-stress-2013-how-environmental-noise-levels-can-spike-your-stress-load

Lindenfeld, G., & Bruursema, L. R. (2015, May 28). *Resetting the Fear Switch in PTSD: A Novel Treatment Using Acoustical Neuromodulation to Modify Memory Reconsolidation.* http://www.academia.edu/12683048/Resetting_the_Fear_Switch_in_PTSD_A_Novel_Treatment_Using_Acoustical_Neuromdulation_to_Modify_Memory_Reconsolidation

Oster, G. (1973). Auditory Beats in the Brain. *Scientific American, 229*(4). http://www.scientificamerican.com/article/auditory-beats-in-the-brain/

Triggers & Flashbacks. (2001, August 7). *University of Alberta Sexual Assault Centre.* Informational. https://www.ualberta.ca/~uasac/Triggers.htm

Veterans_PTSD_BAUD.pdf. http://www.pnpcenter.com/images/Veterans_PTSD_BAUD.pdf

Wagner, K. D. The Science Behind Healing with Sound. *Spirituality & Health.* Informational. http://spiritualityhealth.com/articles/science-behind-healing-sound

Epilogue

Following threat to their survival, numerous species of mammals are inclined to physically and immediately clear the residual effects of the Fight-Flight-Freeze response. Dr. Peter Levine refers to this trauma release mechanism in his writings, as exemplified in a polar bear video. Unfortunately, he perceives that humans: "... no longer know to 'just shake it off' like the polar bear and African deer do innately. We've lost it!" He further suggests that:

"Humans, in contrast to animals, frequently become stuck in a kind of limbo, not fully reengaging in life after experiencing threat as overwhelming terror or horror. In addition, they exhibit a propensity for freezing in situations where a non-traumatized individual might only sense danger or even feel some excitement. Rather than being a last-ditch reaction to inescapable threat, paralysis becomes a 'default' response to a wide variety of situations in which one's feelings are highly aroused." (Levine, 2010)

Dr. Bessel A. Van der Kolk notes that: "Trauma has nothing whatsoever to do with cognition. It has to do with your body being reset to interpret the world as a dangerous place. That reset begins in the deep recesses of the brain with its most primitive structures, regions that no cognitive therapy can access. It's not something you can talk yourself out of." (Kolk, 2015)

Over the course of writing ten chapters pertaining to first responders, it became imminently clear to me that the prior two distinguished authors are absolutely correct in their perspectives. Choosing an occupation that involves random and frequent exposure to trauma appears to have a deleterious effect on those who serve to protect us from harm.

I've written this epilogue as a summary that unifies the clear and predictable consequences of cumulative exposure to the well-being of our service providers. Of course, there are exceptions to this perspective, however, the emergence of awareness related to Delayed Onset PTSD (DOPTSD) among those who have not previously evidenced symptoms may be a forewarning of what is yet to come.

I've highlighted salient points in my review of each chapter, bringing together aspects of compassion fatigue/Post-Traumatic Stress Disorder that likely apply to each of the discussed first responder professions. Fortuitously, Hurricane Irma came into my life causing me and my family to seek shelter at a protected facility.

While there, it came to me that this is where I would come upon first responders, as well as other support entities such as American Red Cross personnel, serving at their finest. This is the ideal we all seek! My goal of ending the nightmare of PTSD among our active duty military and veterans clearly applies to our first responders as well. To assist them to remain at their finest is a noble and achievable goal. I dedicate this book to that purpose.

As noted in Chapter One, the 9/11/01 tragedy served as our wake-up call to the danger and challenges facing us in the twenty-first century. Unfortunately, sixteen years later, we continue to attempt to address this dilemma with methodology that has been proven to be ineffective. We can and must do better than that!

I've estimated that conservatively, 15 to 20% of our first responders are struggling with an active PTSD condition. I vigorously challenged the term 'remitted PTSD', perceiving of this term as an excuse for the inadequacies of current treatments to fully remediate the long-term effects that trauma has on human beings.

Mention was made related to the use of Propranolol to alter the presence of PTSD in our veterans and first responders. The author noted that: "Administration of propranolol prior to or immediately following traumatic situations to prevent emotional memory consolidation may ensure that no traumatic experience becomes embedded in the amygdala as a non-conscious emotional memory." ("Compos Mentis: Undergraduate Journal of Cognition and Neuroethics - cmv2i2.pdf,")

Unbeknown to the author of the article, there is a safe, rapid and non-invasive way to alter the emotional effects of trauma that I call RESET Therapy. This treatment utilizes a special sound to accomplish the removal of the emotional components of trauma without losing the actual memory of the event as suggested through the use of propranolol.

Chapter Two focused on the specialty occupation of policing. I concluded that the longer an officer serves, the more likely he or she is to accumulate the effects of trauma. The 'Thin Blue Line' concept was discussed, with this being based upon the denial of weakness, ridicule of mental infirmities and the 'us against them' philosophy.

The readily available collegial way to cope with the cumulative effects of stress in masculine organizations tends to be through the use of alcohol. This is purported to be able to at least temporarily shield against the impact produced by accumulating trauma. Furthermore, a defense mechanism referred to as 'insulation' further prevents a person from experiencing the awareness of feelings. There is little doubt that this phenomenon further complicates matters among police personnel in their relationship with the communities they serve.

Finally, the topic of health issues consequent to long-term trauma exposure among law enforcement personnel was introduced, including coronary events, digestive disorders, cardiovascular disease, alcoholism, domestic violence, post-traumatic stress disorder, depression, and ultimately suicide.

In Chapter Three, a tendency for weakened resiliency in the aging firefighter was discussed. Frequent exposure to traumatic incidents alters the firefighter's normative sleep patterns. This is further exacerbated by exposure to secondary trauma through critical incident debriefings.

An official position related to Critical Incident Stress Debriefing (CISD) was provided by the U.S. Department of Veterans Affairs – National Center for PTSD advising that: "Available evidence shows that, in some instances, it (CISD) may increase traumatic stress or complicate recovery." ("Types of Debriefing Following Disasters - PTSD,")

Chapter Four (Emergency Medical Services), described the average tenure of EMT personnel as being less than 4 years in duration. This appears to be strongly associated with the number of calls handled by the EMT on a weekly basis.

The quest for the 'ideal' personality type for this occupation is ongoing and from my perspective is fruitless. The impact of cumulative stress and its negative secondary impact on the marital and family relationship appears to be a predictable variable within the context of family stability/instability.

A tendency to avoid seeking professional intervention is clearly a variable among EMT personnel. Apparently, many in this profession choose to leave after a period of four years to seek other employment opportunities. This is a tremendous loss of skill and experience. Finally, the incidence of suicide among EMT personnel tends to be under-reported due to a number of variables.

Chapter Five (Nursing) explored the pressure on nurses' forthcoming from the Affordable Care Act with its associated paperwork and consequent administrative pressure related to increased demand. Long delays in admitting patients places increasing levels of pressure on attending staff, resulting in an escalation in medical errors.

Many perceive that the ER has become a factory assembly line rather than a place of sensitivity and caring that is at the heart of the nursing profession. The term 'boarding' is akin to treating the waiting patient as a product rather than a human being. Alternatively, patient rudeness, unrealistic expectations and demands place ER staff in a precarious position, as they are forced to endure insults as well as risk of violence.

Critical incidents (CI's are also perceived to be a primary problem particularly when demand factors interfere with proper nursing practices. CI's have been defined as events that potentially overwhelm a nurse's usual coping skills and produce unusual distress in a healthy person. I question how long nurses can stay healthy with repeated exposure to CI's throughout the day to day work experience. Issues of miscommunication, burnout, addiction and suicide appear to be an end product resulting from cumulative stress that is so prevalent in this occupation. Are these byproducts also associated with the cumulative number of CI's a nurse is exposed to?

In Chapter Six, the ER Physician began the original journey to licensure through varied 'baptisms of fire' that are apparently thought to wean those who are unable to deal with stress factors. Indeed, the education/ordeal of the doctor appears to be based on numerous and frequent hurdles that test the endurance of the individual rather than ascertain the ability to learn and consequently apply this knowledge in a practical way.

My experience with combat veterans with PTSD is that they are perpetually frozen in the 'protect and defend' mode, having lost growth aspects of their former selves. Might this be the same for the physician who has successfully completed the tribulations of becoming a doctor?

Is it possible that physician "professional burnout," characterized by a loss of enthusiasm for work (emotional exhaustion), feelings of cynicism (depersonalization), etc., are a byproduct of their medical training experience?

I find it quite interesting that among ER doctors, female physicians were substantially more likely to be divorced than males. It has been speculated that the primary variable accounting for this difference is likely attributable to hours worked. Apparently, this is a real difference for the female physician who experiences the dual demands forthcoming from the home and work environment.

I've decided to repeat part of a vignette because it so aptly describes the deteriorating environment in the ER when things begin to systematically go wrong.

"We tend to avoid our everyday stories of insecurity, frustration, and minor irritations. We keep quiet about the shameful bits—forgotten dosages, missed intubations, lost arguments against consultants. We do not talk about second-guessing our career path, missing important deadlines, our rising cholesterol, or an impending divorce." (Chung & MD, 2016)

Is it any wonder that approximately 10% to 12% of physicians develop a substance use disorder during their careers? Note was made that as the physician self-isolates, suicidal ideation accompanies this tendency. It was further speculated that we lose the counterpart of a large medical school class to suicide yearly. This is a ridiculous loss of talented people. We can and must alter these stress related consequences.

Chapter Seven introduces us to the world of the Dispatchers/Telecommunicator. These professionals are the gatekeepers for emergency services provided by police officers, firefighters and paramedics. The ever-developing technology utilized by dispatchers has undoubtedly altered operational efficiency by reducing response time, thereby increasing the number of calls that can be processed per shift. Apparently, what is missing in this matrix is the impact that the increased workload has on the capacity of the human being to interface with potentially traumatic circumstances.

Because the telecommunicator frequently deals with traumatic circumstances, it has long been thought that vicarious trauma might be a byproduct of this exposure. However, when an employee submits a claim for disability consequential to this exposure, the historical 'rule of thumb' was that the claim was denied because the exposure was 'indirect.'

Alteration in the Diagnostic and Statistical Manual of Mental Disorders (DSM-5) related to the criteria necessary for the diagnosis of PTSD occurred in 2015. It is yet to be seen how this impacts future disability claims. If submitted claims are successful, might the 'system' be more amenable to scientifically-based interventions that can remediate the effects of vicarious trauma?

Chapter Eight is focused on the correction officer's responsibilities related to a diverse, at times violent group of incarcerated prisoners. As I described, the prevailing attitude of the correction officer becomes one of 'protect and defend' within the designated work environment.

Indeed, as described, our prison system has become the containment vessel for those in our country with serious mental illness thereby creating an absolute crisis pertaining to this vulnerable population. I was aghast at the incidence of developmental trauma including: "neglect; emotional, physical, and sexual abuse; parental incarceration and binge drinking; and witnessing, being threatened with, and experiencing violence." ("The toll of childhood trauma," 2014)

Furthermore, I found it astounding that over the last 40 years, we have spent trillions of dollars on the failed and ineffective War on Drugs. Another disturbing figure that caught my attention was that about 60 percent of incarcerated adults experienced at least one traumatic brain injury prior to incarceration, thereby consequently costing us around $29,000 a year.

I discussed a recent study that found that PTSD was present in 48% of the prison population. The investigators also found that 70% of imprisoned women experienced childhood sexual abuse with a parallel rate of 50% for men. (Briere et al., 2016)

I've included the previously quoted material in its entirety because I still have a hard time conceiving how someone would enter this profession knowing the following information. "We face some of the ugliest statistics of mortality as correctional officers. Perhaps you have seen these, they are fairly commonly cited online in other articles, but just in case you need a reality check here it is:

- "Correctional Officers (CO's) have the second highest mortality rate of any occupation.
- 33.5% of all assaults in prisons and jails are committed by inmates against staff.
- A CO's 58th birthday, on average, is their last.

- A CO will be seriously assaulted at least twice in a 20-year career.
- On average, a CO will live only 18 months after retirement.
- CO's have a 39% higher suicide rate than any other occupation,
- And have a higher divorce and substance abuse rates then the general population." ("Beating The Odds," 2012)

I believe that we can do better with and for our CO's as well as those who become imprisoned due to earlier trauma exposure. The resources are there. What is lacking is the blueprint and the will to create a change.

Sometimes the whole really is bigger than the sum of its parts. This was the reason that I added Chapter Nine to this book. Our first responders came together during a time of uncertainty. Through the structure they provided, a totally diverse group of frightened people, ridden with doubt about whether they would make it through alive, were able to survive, 'the storm.'

Included in this group were those in nursing homes with serious mental and physical ailments. And yet, we came together as one – looking out for each other. For those with animals, our pets came in all sizes representing the diversity that was reflected in our temporary community.

In retrospect, it was fortuitous for me to have engaged in this experience. There were numerous alternatives available when the order to evacuate was issued. Friends near and far offered shelter. I must tell you that with pets, this certainly was tempting. However, I have learned much of how things can be and am grateful that matters turned out as they did.

I included Chapter Ten because I've alluded to RESET Therapy throughout this text and believed it prudent to provide general information about this intervention. In closing, specifics pertaining to RESET Therapy are available through my varied blogs and books that can be accessed at www.drlindenfeldresettherapy.com. Furthermore, printed versions of my books can be obtained through Amazon.

References

Beating The Odds. http://www.corrections.com/news/article/30096-beating-the-odds

Briere, J., Agee, E., & Dietrich, A. (2016). Cumulative trauma and current post-traumatic stress disorder status in general population and inmate samples. *Psychological Trauma: Theory, Research, Practice and Policy*, *8*(4), 439–446. https://doi.org/10.1037/tra0000107

Chung, A. S., & MD. (2016, August 26). stories to live by. Retrieved November 26, 2016, from https://akosmed.com/2016/08/26/stories-to-live-by/

Compos Mentis: Undergraduate Journal of Cognition and Neuroethics - cmv2i2.pdf. (n.d.). http:// cm.cognethic.org/cmv 2i2.pdf#page=5

Kolk, B. A. V. der. (2015). The Body Keeps the Score: Brain, Mind, and Body in the Healing of Trauma. Penguin Books.

Levine P. A. (2010) In an Unspoken Voice: How the Body Releases Trauma and Restores Goodness. North Atlantic Books.

The toll of childhood trauma. (2014, June 23). https: //ct.counseling.org/2014/06/the-toll-of-childhood-trauma/

Types of Debriefing Following Disasters - PTSD: National Center for PTSD. http://www.ptsd. va.gov/professional/trauma/disaster-terrorism/debriefing-after-disasters.asp